NURTURE EMOTIONAL WELL-BEING FOR WOMEN

EMPOWER YOUR RECOVERY AFTER TRAUMA,
BUILD LASTING RESILIENCE, AND
TRANSFORM PAIN INTO STRENGTH

TERRI STERK

TABLE OF CONTENTS

Introduction   5

1. SOMETHING NEEDS TO CHANGE   13
   What is Trauma?   15
   The Difference Between Complex Post-Traumatic
   Stress Disorder and Post-Traumatic Stress Disorder   21
   Stages of Trauma   22
   Steps in the Healing Process   26
   Interactive Element   29
   Segue   30

2. WHAT HAPPENED TO YOU   31
   Reflect on Your Life Story   33
   What is Narrative Therapy?   36
   Interactive Element   44
   Segue   46

3. KNOCKED DOWN BUT NOT OUT   47
   The Role of Resilience in Healing From Trauma   50
   Practical Resilience Strategies   51
   Interactive Element   58
   Segue   58

4. THE REBUILD BEGINS   59
   Post-Traumatic Growth   61
   Emotional Resilience   63
   Step-By-Step Process for Healing and Growth   69
   Practical Exercises for Your Healing Journey   71
   Interactive Element   74
   Segue   74

5. EMOTIONAL FREEDOM   75
   The Impact of Trauma on Emotional Regulation   77
   The Power of a Thought   86
   Interactive Element   94
   Segue   94

6. COOL, CALM, COLLECTED   97

Emotional Triggers   99

How to Process Emotional Triggers Later   104

Interactive Element   108

Segue   108

7. PROCESSING THE PAST   109

Benefits of Confronting Your Past Traumas   111

Self-Help Therapeutic Techniques   118

Guidance to Find Help From Mental Health
Practitioners   125

Interactive Element   127

8. STAND IN YOUR POWER   129

Personal Empowerment   131

Who Do You Tell?   136

Self-Advocacy   138

Interactive Element   143

Segue   144

9. A VISION OF SOMETHING BETTER   145

Build a Meaningful Life   147

Why We Need Hope and How to Create It   149

How to Achieve Goals   151

Interactive Element   152

Segue   152

10. BUILDING ON YOUR FOUNDATIONS   153

The Significance of Building a Support Network   156

The Relationship Between Self-Care and Healing   157

How to Increase Personal Growth   161

Interactive Element   163

Segue   163

Conclusion   165

References   171

INTRODUCTION

Healing doesn't mean the pain never existed. It means the damage no longer controls our lives. — NotSalmon.com

History and society have a toxic trend of trying to pretend trauma does not exist. However, it does, and unresolved trauma is messing up our lives. You may already notice its impact on your life, or perhaps you are still sitting with unresolved questions. By deciding to heal your trauma, you take a courageous, positive step in the right direction to find the quality of life you deserve. Platitudes, toxic positivity, and glib phrases are used to shut you up or make the "problem" disappear:

- "It's in the past; just move on."
- "You should be over it by now."
- "You're too sensitive."
- "Other people have it worse."

- "You're just seeking attention or excuses."
- "You should forgive and forget."
- "Are you sure it really happened?"
- "What is wrong with you?"

When you are already struggling with trauma, further reactions and lack of support can leave you doubting yourself and your sanity. As you read this book, here are the baseline facts to remember:

- Suppose you find yourself grappling with emotional regulation, frequent triggers, or feelings of stress, anxiety, fear, or depression. In that case, issues from your past are likely impacting your present. Addressing these issues can significantly ease the challenges you face.
- If you cannot enjoy a calm, mostly happy, and stable existence and the effects of the past remain with you, it means you need help and support, not criticism and useless platitudes.
- No matter the nature of the event or how others perceive it if recalling it evokes feelings of sadness, fear, or discomfort, it could indicate you may be carrying unresolved trauma.

Never let anyone tell you what you should think or feel. Don't dismiss bad feelings because that is just "kicking the can" down the road. If you read this book, you are likely struggling with questions or looking for a deeper understanding of yourself and your circumstances. Remember, your journey is unique, and only you have the power to define your path. You, too, are worth the effort of finding it.

Over the past twenty years, my life has been a compilation of traumatic events, each a piece of a puzzle that now interlocks to form the collage of my life. In 2003, I was diagnosed with breast cancer. This shocking revelation coincided with my 40th birthday while my children were still young. Tragedy struck again in 2006 when we lost a family member who took his own life.

In 2011, my world was shaken once more when my mother passed away unexpectedly after a brief illness. That same year, I was displaced from my job of 20 years. Two years later, in 2013, I received my second diagnosis of breast cancer. Then, 2015 was marked by the loss of my father after progressive dementia and mobility loss. One year later, in 2016, a dear friend lost her life after metastatic breast cancer. In 2017, my family experienced the death of my mother-in-law after a long illness. I also experienced another job loss, as well as unhealed family estrangement that persists to the current day.

These events left me questioning what was next for me. The chronic stress and emotional strain left me struggling to heal. The unhealed pain blocked any effort I made to move forward.

Looking back, I see the people who surrounded my family and me during these challenging times. I started a gratefulness journal to recognize all the goodness in my life, which has helped me see the blessings in my past experiences. I discovered gratitude for the relationships built on love and kindness, the compassion my children learned, the steadfast support from my husband, and the extra time with my dad during his final months. With the gift of time to nurture my body, mind, and spirit, I am now grounded with peace and calm. The gratefulness journal was the tipping point to help me jumpstart my healing journey. I now embrace a sense of well-being and good health that I didn't even know was possible. I had to start somewhere.

You may have had your memories and trauma glossed over, ignored, dismissed, or diminished by people who should have stepped in and helped you. It may have taken you a long time to realize that what happened was intrinsically wrong, that you are worth more, and that your support systems and society have somewhat failed you. You may have struggled with the fallout of the trauma while feeling bad, guilty, and somehow broken. People's reactions to your distress have not generally been helpful and often made the pain worse. As a survivor of trauma, you frequently grapple with intense emotional distress, including feelings of sadness, anxiety, anger, guilt, shame, and fear. These overwhelming emotions will interfere with your daily life. You might experience distressing flashbacks and intrusive memories related to traumatic events. These are highly distressing and disruptive, causing you to relive the trauma.

Trauma impacts your ability to form and maintain healthy relationships. It becomes a struggle to trust others, creating interpersonal conflicts and difficulty forming attachments.Trauma erodes your self-esteem and self-worth. You may struggle with inadequacy, self-blame, and a negative self-image. Unresolved trauma manifests in physical symptoms such as chronic pain, sleep disturbances, and other health problems. These physical manifestations can add to your overall distress and discomfort.

Since you are still reading, you are likely at a point where you wish to be carefree and feel complete inner peace without the strain and stain of the trauma on your life. As much as you want a genie to grant you three wishes, it's impossible. Trauma cannot be dissipated by wishing or pushing it away. This book, *Nurture Emotional Well-*

Being for Women, is your ticket to achieving the life you wish you had. Through exploring the essence of emotional resilience, you will learn the art of self-advocacy and discover the power of positive psychology. This book offers practical strategies to regain your inner equilibrium and transform pain into unwavering strength. If you are ready and willing to do the work, this book holds the following benefits:

- **Increased understanding:** Deepen your knowledge of trauma, how it personally affects you, and the factors that contribute to your emotional and psychological challenges.
- **Emotional regulation:** Learn what it means to heal trauma and use the strategies and techniques taught by trauma-informed therapists to gain better control of your emotional response.
- **Improved coping skills:** Develop new coping skills and strategies to deal with triggers, flashbacks, and other distressing symptoms.
- **Resilience building:** Cultivate the strength and resilience needed to face life's challenges.
- **Healthy relationships:** Improve your ability to form and maintain healthy relationships through better communication, trust, and intimacy.
- **Increased self-compassion:** Nurture a more supportive relationship with yourself by diminishing self-criticism and self-blame.
- **Empowerment:** Find hope and motivation to take control of your healing journey with relatable stories of survivors who have healed from trauma.
- **Better self-management:** Learn to set boundaries, prioritize self-care, and manage stress more effectively, contributing to a healthier and more balanced life.

- **Integration of trauma experiences:** Acquire knowledge to use your pain to find meaning and purpose in your healing journey by integrating your traumatic experiences into your life story.
- **Lifestyle changes:** Feel motivated to make positive changes, such as adopting healthier habits, seeking therapy or support groups, and prioritizing your mental and emotional well-being.
- **Increased advocacy and support:** Become an advocate for yourself and others who have experienced trauma to provide support and resources to others in need.

"Nurture Emotional Well-Being for Women" presents a rebuilding and resiliency blueprint tailored to assist women who have endured challenging experiences to reclaim their inner balance and strength. It guides readers to advocate for themselves, articulate their needs and rights, and reconstruct a more resilient life. Using cognitive therapy and a modern behavioral support map, it takes you through a process using practical tools and methods that will each have a positive ripple effect.

Along with the book, you also have access to the Free Interactive Elements Workbook, which supplements each chapter with worksheets for applying the concepts discussed.

Use this QR Code to access the workbook.

By the end of the book, you can expect significant changes in your state of mind and external life. Empower your recovery by building lasting resilience, restoring inner balance, and using your pain to find newfound strength.

It's important to note that the healing process from trauma is highly individual, and not everyone will experience the same outcomes. Progress may be gradual and may involve setbacks along the way.

One in three women will experience some form of traumatic life experience that needs recognition and support. The vital skills shared in this book will guide you on a transformative journey from enduring pain to reclaiming control over your life, harnessing your power and peace of mind.

Please contact me with any questions. I'm cheering you on!

Terri Sterk

tsterkemotionalhealing@gmail.com

1

SOMETHING NEEDS TO CHANGE

> *We cannot change anything until we accept it.*
> *Condemnation does not liberate, it oppresses.*
>
> — CARL JUNG

O ften, a tragic life event makes you realize something needs to change. Dawne shared her inspirational story of how her life changed after a horrific car crash (Trauma Survivor's Network, n.d.):

One week before Dawne's crash, she was on vacation in Florida with her boyfriend. Suddenly awakened in the middle of the night, Dawne experienced an overwhelming premonition of impending tragedy. Recounting the eerie sensation, she recalls, "I thought I was going to get a call that someone had passed unexpectedly."

Reflecting on the persistent unease that lingered for days, Dawne couldn't shake the unsettling, anxious feeling. A week later, fate dealt a devastating blow as she became involved in a horrific car crash while making a left-hand turn on her way to work. Transported initially to a local hospital, the severity of her injuries necessitated a transfer to a trauma hospital, where she grappled with multiple injuries, including a head injury and a harrowing seatbelt wound.

Dawne spent three days in the trauma unit and was also unable to walk. She vividly remembers the mixed emotions of anticipation and fear as she prepared to leave the hospital. "I was excited to be leaving and couldn't wait to shower, wash my hair, and put on my pajamas," she recalls. However, the reality of post-crash life hit hard —terrifying experiences in vehicles, unanticipated pain after the morphine wore off, and the harsh adjustment to a new normal dominated by daily medical care.

Navigating the aftermath involved grappling with financial strain, flashbacks, sleepless nights, and persistent anxiety. Dawne's once-beloved job and social life abruptly stopped, revealing the true colors of her friendships. "I realized who my true friends were when those I thought would show up were suddenly unavailable."

Embarking on a formidable learning curve and recovery process, Dawne's crash in 2012 marked the beginning of a journey that continues today. Enduring chronic pain, sleepless nights, and flashbacks, she remained committed in 2016 to her rehabilitation. Dawne took a proactive step by establishing an online support group for Motor Vehicle Crash Survivors, recognizing the need for post-hospitalization assistance. "Knowing you are not alone can save you, and bringing crash survivors together to find support in one another is very therapeutic," she affirms.

Peering into the rear-view mirror of that fateful morning, Dawne sees the evolution from fear to courage, helplessness to independence, and weakness to strength. Professional strangers from the medical and legal realms have transformed into lasting friends, shaping Dawne's life for years. Through her struggles, she discovered the absence of available post-discharge support, prompting her to create an online medium that now connects over 700 members—individuals either recovering from their crashes or just beginning their journey. Dawne's resilience has made her experience a beacon of hope for others facing similar challenges.

Dawne used a traumatic incident and turned it into something positive that benefits the well-being of others. In this opening chapter, you can recognize your life's need for healing and transformation and gain insight into the impact of trauma and its implications on your well-being.

This chapter aims to bring you to a turning point in your healing journey. You have the opportunity to understand the importance of healing from trauma at an early stage because trauma has long-term effects on your overall well-being.

WHAT IS TRAUMA?

In professional terms, trauma would be described as an experience that overwhelms the nervous system and leaves the brain to handle the situation. Still, the brain then realizes it lacks the coping skills to handle the trauma. The experience starts to live in the body, which leaves emotional scars and a distressing memory that creeps up unexpectedly and manifests in various unwanted ways. If left unresolved, you risk the potential of developing post-traumatic stress disorder (PTSD).

Trauma is a personal experience, and only you have the power to define an experience as traumatic. You can't fully grasp the impact of a traumatic event when you're in the heat of the moment. Under immense stress, you go into "survival mode." Your sympathetic nervous system prepares your body for stressful or dangerous situations. It kicks in, and you operate on an evolutionary instinct to either stay and fight, flee to save yourself or freeze.

After I finished my breast cancer treatment, others made me feel like I was doing well and just fine to move on. In reality, I was not physically or mentally prepared.

No one can tell you the extent of your traumatic experience. Many people do not know how to respond when you tell them about your experience. To soothe themselves, they tend to minimize or invalidate your feelings by saying, "It's not that bad," or "That's not how it happened."

Your experience is uniquely your own; only you get to say what you need or what is not working for you. If the traumatic event psychologically impacted you, it means it was terrible for you. Our resilience levels and personalities differ, and our responses might vary for the same type of stress. The differences are entirely normal and okay. No matter your story, it's understandable if you've only recently realized you're ready to confront your past and the negative impacts of the trauma on your current life.

Different Types of Trauma

Trauma can be a one-time or an ongoing experience. In many cases, you experience traumatic events but often fail to see them as such. This section will clear up any uncertainty of what incidents have the potential to cause trauma.

Physical abuse occurs when someone violates your body and disrespects your physical boundaries. Physical abuse is a traumatizing event that leads to feeling uncomfortable in your own body or avoiding any type of physical contact with others. For example, Lexi was on her way to buy lunch on her break when a random guy who walked past her touched her inappropriately and then laughed about it. Lexi was angry at herself for not retaliating in the moment. This traumatic event made her change her fashion sense, and she started to refrain from hugging male family members and friends.

Verbal abuse is seen as a type of emotional abuse that occurs when someone says hurtful things to you that leave an emotional scar. Being bullied by a boss or friend, parents making hurtful and cruel comments, and your partner calling you names are all different ways emotional abuse can traumatize you. Martha was bullied at school from a young age, never told anybody, and developed into an adult with extremely low self-esteem.

In Martha's early twenties, she met Stefan, who she believed was the love of her life. He constantly yelled at her, questioned everything she did, called her names in the presence of her friends and belittled her every chance he got. Martha ended up with a fragile ego, became hypersensitive to criticism, and was later diagnosed with chronic anxiety.

Childhood traumas are vastly underestimated as you may fail to see how much they have shaped you as an adult. One form of childhood trauma worth exploring is childhood neglect. Your parents may have been in your life daily, but were they able to successfully fulfill all your needs as a child? Neglect in childhood is defined as your parent's inability to meet your emotional and physical needs.

Physical demands refer to feeding, bathing, providing safe and clean housing, and securing medical care. Emotional needs are explained as a parent comforting you when you are emotionally distressed. Neglect of emotional support as a child significantly influences your relationships as an adult. It impacts how you express and regulate your emotions. Rachel chronicles her story of childhood emotional neglect.

As a young girl, Rachel had a heart filled with innocence and a deep care for all creatures. One day, a family friend gifted them a cat named Momma Cat, a lovely outdoor feline seeking a new home.

During breakfast, Rachel saved some bacon fat to feed Momma Cat, venturing outside in her nightgown to offer the treat. Unexpectedly, the cat bit her, leading to a moment of pain and shock as blood trickled down her hand. Hearing her cries, Rachel's father swiftly intervened, shooting Momma Cat in a moment of panic and protection.

The traumatic incident left Rachel scarred, with her older sister unfairly blaming her for the cat's fate. Rachel buried the memory deep within, growing introverted and shy as she navigated through life.

Years passed, bringing milestones like high school graduation and her parents' separation. A casual day at the mall with her mother and sister unexpectedly resurfaced memories of the farm days, including the tragic incident with Momma Cat. In a crowded food court, the weight of the suppressed memory hit Rachel hard, triggering a flood of emotions and tears, releasing years of pent-up guilt and sorrow.

Reflecting on the painful memory, Rachel realized how it had shaped her perspective and behavior over the years. The incident's impact lingered within her, influencing her interactions and choices and highlighting the need for healing and understanding as she navigated the complexities of her past.

"A year later, I found the courage to ask my dad about the incident," Rachel shared. His explanation that it was a lesson about life and death did little to ease her pain or confusion. Growing up on a farm,

Rachel knew all too well about the cycle of life, but the sudden and violent nature of Momma Cat's demise had left a deep scar on her young heart.

The realization that her past trauma still held power over her present and future led Rachel to consider seeking help to navigate the complex emotions and find a path toward healing and forgiveness. Rachel embarked on a journey of self-discovery and healing, recognizing that the road to forgiveness and inner peace would require courage, vulnerability, and a willingness to confront the shadows of the past.

"The scars of the past may never fully fade," Rachel reflected. With the support of her therapist, she embarked on a healing journey that would lead her to forgiveness and acceptance. Rachel discovered a newfound sense of purpose and clarity, paving the way for a brighter, more empowered future filled with hope and possibility.

If you experienced trauma during your childhood, the experience may have had adverse effects on your overall well-being, growth, and development. Trauma can alter the growth of your brain, which causes trouble with controlling emotions. Traumatized children have a sense of fear within them, which constantly sets off their body's stress alarm. Your childhood experiences that didn't scare other children your age might have caused you intense distress. You might still struggle to identify and control your emotions as an adult. It is essential in trauma recovery to develop the skills to regulate your emotions so you can stay calm during the storm.

Let's continue the discussion of the different types of trauma.

Persistent low-grade stress is an underrated form of trauma of constantly being in a stressful environment. Stress can result from various parts of your life, including your job, family dynamics, abusive relationships, or the community in which you live. You might not recognize each situation as traumatic. Still, small or minor stressful incidents experienced over time will create difficult emotions.

Severely stressful incidents can precipitate the onset of acute stress disorder or post-traumatic stress disorder (PTSD). Nicole resides in a community characterized by a high crime rate. Random shootings, violent altercations among community members, and numerous homicides within the two months since Nicole moved into the neighborhood have created an atmosphere of fear. Nicole harbors constant anxiety, mainly when leaving her house, stemming from the day she witnessed a six-year-old boy being shot a short distance away. Living with undiagnosed PTSD, Nicole has come to accept her challenging circumstances.

Other types of traumas include: (Mitts, n.d.)

- Suffering grief due to the sudden death of a loved one,
- Divorce or other intense break-up,
- Observing a violent incident,
- Experiencing mistreatment or harm from religious practices,
- Witnessing or enduring domestic abuse,
- Encountering a physical or emotional assault,
- Withstanding a significant or major accident,
- Impacted by a natural disaster,
- Confronted with a diagnosis of cancer or a chronic illness,
- Facing estrangement from adult children, parents, or siblings.

As stated earlier, the depth of your traumatic experience cannot be accurately conveyed by others. So, you may have additional experiences to add to the list.

THE DIFFERENCE BETWEEN COMPLEX POST-TRAUMATIC STRESS DISORDER AND POST-TRAUMATIC STRESS DISORDER

Post-traumatic stress disorder (PTSD) is a common mental health condition that has been widely used in society. It's normal to temporarily struggle with adjusting or coping with life after a traumatic event. You may be developing PTSD when it comes to a point where the impact of the trauma intensifies, lasts for an extended time frame, and negatively affects your ability to function.

You can recognize symptoms of PTSD if you have intrusive memories about a traumatic event, you avoid anything that triggers you, and you notice an adverse change in your mood, thinking style, and reactions. Experiencing a traumatic event doesn't necessarily mean that you will develop PTSD. You are at risk of developing PTSD after a traumatic event if you also:

- Lack of a support system,
- Have experienced trauma in the past,
- Are diagnosed with anxiety or depression,
- Have a predisposition for anxiety or depression,
- Experience other stressors at the time,
- Struggle to regulate your body's response to intense stress.

Complex PTSD (CPTSD) is somewhat different from PTSD, although they share many of the same symptoms. So, what is complex PTSD (CPTSD), and how does it differ from PTSD? CPTSD is a variation of PTSD in which you experience a few of the same symptoms along with finding it difficult to cope with your emotions and maintain relationships. Symptoms you will experience when developing CPTSD include feeling shame and worthlessness, being unable to effectively control your emotional reactions, struggling to connect with others, and having difficulty developing and sustaining relationships. CPTSD may arise for many reasons, such as:

- Suffering from childhood trauma,
- Enduring abuse in the past or present,
- Escaping the trauma was difficult,
- Experiencing harm by a trusted person.

STAGES OF TRAUMA

From the moment you encounter the traumatic event, you are experiencing one of the stages of trauma. Understanding the five stages of trauma helps you manage the aftermath of the traumatizing event and might prevent PTSD from developing.

Next, the five stages of trauma are explained:

1. **Denial** involves protecting yourself by denying the reality of what has happened. You may minimize the event's intensity by convincing yourself and others that what happened wasn't *that* bad.
2. **Anger** leaves you prepared to release the defense mechanism of denial and transition into a phase where you begin to confront the reality of the event. In this stage, you become angry about what happened. But understand that experiencing intense animosity after trauma is a normal reaction. Allow your rage to exist without shaming

yourself. Anger is another defense mechanism where you hide the emotions you are experiencing toward the traumatic event. For example, instead of being sad, you express anger to mask the sadness.

3. **Bargaining** occurs after you work through stages one and two when you begin to release defense mechanisms and have the strength to take control. An example of bargaining is thinking of the "what ifs" or asking your higher power to erase the traumatic event from your life. For instance, Sara lost her four-month-old baby to brain cancer, and every day, she prayed for God to bring her baby back. Bargaining is another way of delaying the reality of facing what happened.

4. **Depression** results after stages two and three when you are highly charged with emotions and actively want to control what has happened to you. In stage four, you become sad as a result of the pain and loss that comes with trauma. You start to feel empty and hopeless, lose interest in your favorite activities, have low energy, and develop bad sleep habits.

5. **Acceptance** is the final stage in which you feel you are in a space where you can acknowledge what happened and are ready to heal. Acceptance means you embrace the traumatic event for what it is and make peace with how it changed you. You reach this stage when you feel intellectually and emotionally ready to deal with the emotions and aftermath of the traumatic event.

It is important to note that in some situations, these stages may occur in any order and even revert to previously experienced stages. Also, many people miss going through the stages. Instead, they choose to sweep their trauma under the rug and move on as if it never happened. Unfortunately, trauma doesn't magically disappear from your life. You may pretend like the trauma never happened, but it will change you in ways that are unhealthy for your well-being.

When you suppress trauma, your mind and body become stuck in the past. You hope that the trauma is suppressed so far down that it doesn't come back to bite you. Unresolved trauma creeps up on you in the most unexpected times through your physical and emotional reactions. Though the traumatic incident happened months or years ago, your present circumstances will still be impacted by the past.

Unprocessed and unresolved trauma causes your view of the world to be tainted. Your past may impact every new experience. You cannot simply enjoy a moment or experience life in the present, as the unresolved trauma reminds you of what happened in the past. You become defensive and protective of yourself as a coping skill because, ultimately, you are living life as if the traumatic incident occurred a few seconds ago. Unresolved trauma makes you an extremely hypervigilant person—you are always on the lookout for threats. Unresolved trauma can make you fall into substance abuse or other unhealthy coping techniques to manage the symptoms of unprocessed emotions.

I can tell you from my experience unresolved trauma will seek redemption. I began to interpret the actions of others as harmful or threatening, which led to broken relationships.

I lost my mom in 2011 after a grueling three-week hospital stay. It was unexpected and heart-wrenching for the whole family. After the death of my mom, I jumped head-first with my family into care-giving for my father, who was dealing with dementia and declining mobility.

In 2013, I was diagnosed with breast cancer for the second time. So, I jumped again, this time back into the cancer underworld, as I called it. I had been in this place before, ten years earlier, with my first diagnosis. This time, I dealt with more than 18 months of surgeries and chemotherapy while also spending time helping my dad as much as possible.

When I lost my dad in 2015, my emotional state was in a dark place. My support system disappeared, so I faked it to get through day-to-day life. I was too proud to ask for help. All of the losses I had experienced in those five years left me spiraling to find a way to move forward. I was physically exhausted and emotionally drained. After years of repressing my feelings, I couldn't even feel them anymore. Yet I knew something was wrong. I was numb, depressed, and anxious all at the same time.

Grief is complex and not a linear process; it can resurface unexpectedly and be triggered by events, other traumas, people, or many other circumstances. In 2016, I lost my dear friend, Lauren, to metastatic breast cancer.

I was left with survivor's guilt after Lauren's death. This complex emotion can arise after surviving a traumatic event when others did not, leading to feelings of guilt, shame, and self-blame. Lauren was one of my closest friends. She was diagnosed with breast cancer about three years after me. Her diagnosis was changed to stage 4 when it became metastatic. After a 10-year dance with what she affectionately called "armpit cancer," we lost Lauren to her disease.

Survivor's guilt can feel overwhelming at times, but it is not uncommon to feel this way after you have survived a traumatic or difficult life event. Acknowledging your guilt and getting help if these feelings become too difficult to manage alone is vital.

With the help of my spiritual lay minister, I eventually recognized unresolved grief was showing up in many ways. My healing needs became ever-present over time. I realized I had never processed and healed after the death of my mother in 2011. Grief can present differently in many of us; it's a unique and multifaceted experience. Moving through grief is a very personal journey.

Societal expectations, cultural norms, and individual factors such as coping mechanisms or past experiences might hinder the grieving process. I experienced this firsthand when healing from my traumas.

The trauma healing process doesn't just go away, never to be seen again. Still, it does get more manageable and less triggering. Learning to cope and heal from trauma is our next topic.

STEPS IN THE HEALING PROCESS

Carl Jung's quote at the beginning of this chapter is an insightful statement about the nature of change and acceptance.

> *We cannot change anything until we accept it. Condemnation does not liberate, it oppresses.*
>
> — CARL JUNG

The first step toward any form of transformation is acceptance of a situation, a person, or oneself. Without acceptance, we remain stuck in a cycle of denial and resistance, which hinders our ability to move forward. Conversely, condemnation is a form of judgment that only oppresses and limits our potential. It creates a barrier that prevents us from seeing the possibilities for change and growth. Therefore, to truly liberate ourselves and initiate change, we must first embrace acceptance and let go of condemnation.

> *Trauma creates change you don't choose. Healing is about creating the change you do choose.*
>
> — MICHELLE ROSENTHAL

Healing from your trauma is to live in the present without allowing it to be impacted by your past. You can live life freely without the emotional and mental burden of your trauma.

The debate has been ongoing on whether revisiting and discussing the traumatic event could result in healing or destruction. Healing is a personal experience; what works for you may not work for another. Some trauma survivors find peace and healing from telling and retelling their experiences. In contrast, others find it destructive to speak about their trauma and claim that it takes a significant toll on their well-being.

Do you feel it would be beneficial to revisit the traumatic memories while on your healing journey?

If so, let's review the steps below.

The first step to healing from trauma is to create a sense of safety, which may mean finding a quiet spot to sit and reflect on your feelings. Once you feel comfortable and safe in your body, you can move to the second step in the healing process.

The second step requires you to talk or write about the trauma you have experienced, to allow all emotions to be felt, and to try to make meaning of it. You could discuss your memories with a trusted family member, friend, faith representative, or therapist. Or write it out in a journal.

The last step focuses on not letting the circumstances that happened to you define you. Instead, you will create a new sense of self and integrate the traumatic event into your life story. You also start to feel empowered and ready to face life again. You will choose the healing.

Knowing When to Seek Help for Trauma

No matter where you are in your journey of healing from trauma, it's crucial to recognize when your symptoms become too much to handle, start interfering with your daily life, or feel unmanageable. If you are experiencing trauma symptoms that have persisted for more than one month without improvement, seeking support from a medical professional or mental health expert is advisable. These trained professionals can help you address and manage these challenges effectively so you can get back to creating a life you love.

Embracing the unique nature of the healing journey is paramount, recognizing that each individual's path is personal and unfolds at its own pace. Strive to liberate yourself from the confines of impractical timelines, granting the necessary time and space for the healing process. The following strategies, adapted from insights by Gillette (2022), can prove instrumental in navigating intense emotions:

- **Promptly Acknowledge Emotions:** Identify and label your feelings as they surface, fostering a heightened self-awareness that serves as the foundation for healing.
- **Cultivate Mindfulness:** Engage in activities that focus your mind on the present moment. These activities can

offer a respite from overwhelming emotions and promote a sense of inner calm.

- **Foster Laughter and Joy:** Incorporate activities that bring genuine humor and delight into your routine. Laughter can be a powerful antidote to emotional distress.
- **Enhance Lifestyle Practices:** Commit to improving your overall lifestyle, encompassing aspects such as physical activity, nutrition, and sleep, as these play integral roles in supporting emotional well-being.
- **Reach Out for Support:** Seek assistance and guidance from mental health professionals or trusted individuals. Recognize the strength in sharing your struggles and receiving support.
- **Avoid False Narratives:** Resist the temptation to construct inaccurate narratives surrounding the traumatic event, allowing for a more objective and realistic understanding of the experience.

By incorporating these strategies into your healing journey, you empower yourself with practical tools to navigate the complexities of intense emotions while fostering a compassionate and self-affirming approach to personal recovery.

INTERACTIVE ELEMENT

The Chapter 1 Trauma Self-Assessment Quiz is in the Free Interactive Elements Workbook. You will reflect and respond to the questions to determine whether you have experienced trauma and need healing.

Use the QR code below to access the documents.

SEGUE

This chapter sets the stage for creating a healing journey. First, consider how your trauma story has shaped your current outlook to move toward healing. Then, in Chapter 2, we will discuss rebuilding and changing the narrative of your trauma story to support the life you want. In the following chapters, we will delve deeper into understanding what has happened and how to initiate the healing process.

2

WHAT HAPPENED TO YOU

> *The paradox of trauma is that it has both the power to destroy and the power to transform and resurrect.*
>
> — PETER A. LEVINE

The quote is factual about the impact trauma may have on you. Trauma can shatter your world into pieces and completely change your life. Still, it can bring growth, personal development, and positive change. If you are ready to share your story, you are prepared to embark on your healing journey. Each chapter of this book is sprinkled with stories from trauma thrivers in various stages of their journeys. Hearing other people's stories can help you overcome fear or anxiety about telling your story.

May you find peace, perspective, inspiration, and courage in these stories.

Sammy, once a devoted stay-at-home mom and wife, found herself thrust into unexpected turmoil when her husband, John, who had treated her like a queen, confessed to infidelity and requested a divorce. This abrupt revelation marked a profound turning point in Sammy's life, a shift she had never anticipated. Suddenly transformed into a single mother, Sammy moved back in with her parents and faced unemployment, grappling with the unexpected challenges life had thrown her way.

The emotional toll was significant, leading Sammy through episodes of depression and uncertainty about her future. During a particularly dark period, she attempted to take her own life twice. During this bleak phase, Sammy's mother, offering tough love and honesty, implored her to "Get yourself together, Sammy." This candid conversation served as a catalyst, prompting Sammy to realize the need to take control of her life.

Motivated by the desire to overcome her divorce, Sammy initiated a remarkable transformation. Securing a retail job, she pursued part-time studies to become a teacher while dedicated to raising her two children. Observers were astounded by Sammy's newfound drive and accomplishments, prompting many friends to inquire, "What happened to you?" They marveled at her resilience and determination in pursuing her goals.

In this chapter, readers are encouraged to delve into their personal trauma narratives, contemplating how these experiences have molded their lives. The crucial question arises: Did your trauma shatter your existence, become a catalyst for positive transformation, or is the outcome still unclear? Additionally, the chapter explores the therapeutic benefits of narrative therapy, shedding light on its role in facilitating healing from traumatic experiences.

REFLECT ON YOUR LIFE STORY

Your life story starts the day you were born. Every person has a life story that consists of significant and specific stories. Reminiscing your life story reminds you of how far you have come, what you have experienced, and how much you have endured. Your life story plays a role in the person you are today. All life experiences molded your identity, personality, and worldview.

Not everyone is eager to share their trauma or to reflect on what caused their trauma. Reflecting on your story brings back unwanted feelings and memories that are difficult to manage. Parts of your life story may make you feel ashamed or proud; other parts you wish had never happened. This process is often called the "work" as it can sometimes be tricky, even arduous. However, it is through this "work" that warriors are made.

Tammy describes her life as full of "insane twists and turns." She says, "Tragedy equals pain, and then it turns into a crazy miracle."

Tammy was left alone with two children when her husband Eric died after a massive heart attack at home while getting ready for work. Their focus had been on Tammy, who was dealing with stage 4 breast cancer. "We were ill-prepared, and I don't want that to happen again. So, I've done so much in the last six years since losing my husband, figuring out how to feed my children from the grave. I've learned warriors are not born. We are made, and the materials used to make us are pain, suffering, and agony."

Tammy's husband had served in their city Police Department for roughly 27 years, earning a retirement package with the promise of ongoing health care for his family. It was supposed to carry them through after the time of his death until Tammy reached 65 and their two children grew up. Dependent on Eric's health insurance from his police detective career, Tammy was left fighting a loophole that left her without health coverage for herself and her children. With the help of ABC News, she secured coverage and shed light on the dilemma for herself and others who may live the same fate.

Tammy's focus now is leaving a legacy for her children. She is using Facebook to chronicle her story with photos and narrative. With strong faith, she finds the positive in every situation. "I'm still appreciative of being able to wake up every day and do anything I wish. I am also grateful to speak on the phone and see my beautiful children's faces. I am thankful I have a roof over my head, food in my stomach, and many other simple things that most people may take for granted."

Reflecting on your life story and identifying traumatic experiences can provide answers and realizations needed to enhance your overall well-being. Reflecting on your life story initiates a journey down memory lane, where you revisit cherished moments with all of your heart and confront negative memories that stir discomfort deep within you. Do not sugarcoat or tell a watered-down version to please others when reflecting on your story. This reflection is just for you. It's your truth and healing. Be strong and practice healthy ways to self-soothe while looking at your life story.

Self-Soothing Techniques

Be prepared with this list of suggestions for self-soothing techniques before you embark on your healing journey. Pain from recalling these traumatic experiences will catch you off guard if you aren't prepared for them. Consider keeping these health-focused self-soothing ideas in your warrior handbag.

- Take a deep breath and slowly release it through pursed lips.
- Ground yourself using a quick meditation.
- Listen to your favorite song; hum a sound or melody.
- Watch a funny video.
- Take a cold shower or splash cold water over your face.
- Enjoy self-massage of your neck, shoulders, or feet.
- Snuggle or play with your pet.
- Play with a stress-relief toy (fidget spinner, stress ball, Rubik's cube).
- Try the Emotional Freedom Technique (EFT) or tapping.
- Step outside to breathe fresh air and enjoy the sunshine for a few minutes.
- Close your eyes, feel the breeze, and listen to the sounds around you.
- Go for a meandering walk and notice the little things you usually would zip past.
- Take yourself out for coffee or tea.
- Eat some dark chocolate.
- Slowly and intentionally cook a meal.
- Take three deep breaths before eating a meal or snack.
- Sniff a lovely scent.
- Move your body; relax your muscles.
- Do lunges or squats to move energy quickly.
- Connect with a friend, deeply or lightheartedly, whichever you are craving.
- Write about your emotions in your journal.

Most of these techniques focus on soothing your nervous system, providing your body with whatever it's lacking, and shifting your emotions to a balanced and happier emotional state. Focus on the feelings coming up in your body. Where is it located? What does it feel like? Your go-to soothing technique may vary from day to day, depending on what sensations arise. Trusting and interpreting your body's communication style plays a significant role in healing trauma.

Before you even start writing your story, consider playing around with self-soothing. When uncomfortable feelings arise, what can you do to show yourself some love? In a given moment, what could work right now? A quick neck massage, deep breaths, or you may have time to call a friend. After experiencing several of these techniques, a list of favorites will likely begin to form. These will become your go-to strategies for bringing love and attention inward, anytime and anywhere.

WHAT IS NARRATIVE THERAPY?

Consider the story of Lori, a 30-year-old female who reaped the benefits of narrative therapy (Expressions Counseling, n.d.).

Lori was dealing with a broken heart and experienced challenging, intense emotions and overwhelming feelings. She had trouble eating and sleeping and stopped taking care of herself. Lori felt lost and did not know who she was without her ex-partner.

In total, she attended eight therapy sessions, during which they conducted a personal assessment and allowed Lori to reflect on her story. As she told her story about how the break-up occurred, she also unpacked her emotions toward the situation. Lori's therapist suggested mindfulness techniques to encourage her to engage in self-care and help her become aware of her emotional reactions and triggers. Lori was encouraged to express her emotions; she chose to journal as a safe outlet.

Narrative therapy made Lori comfortable with facing intense feelings about the breakup. The experience later focused her attention on building an identity that is unique and independent from her previous romantic relationship. In addition, Lori has become a more confident woman as she engages in activities she used to enjoy and has started to pursue her personal goals.

Narrative therapy guides individuals through the healing journey and the pursuit of personal development goals. Central to this approach is exploring how trauma communicates through one's narrative. Inner voices are powerful, and sharing a story can help individuals use more empowering language and veer away from negative self-talk. Trauma can manifest in various ways, leading to different stories influenced by the audience, the individual's current emotional state, and their stage in the healing process.

By delving into these narratives, individuals can gain insight into the impact of trauma on their lives and relationships. Through rewriting and reframing these stories, narrative therapy empowers individuals to separate themselves from the grip of trauma and craft new narratives that foster healing, resilience, and personal growth. This intentional reshaping of life stories paves the way for transformative healing and cultivating a more empowered sense of self.

The way we narrate our lives can significantly shape our identity and perspectives. Think about it. If our words and thoughts are constantly repeating mantras like, "I suck at this" or "I caused this," then those patterns will keep showing up in our lives. A self-blaming or negatively framed story keeps one closely tied to that narrative. Narrative therapy empowers by highlighting that individuals are not defined by their stories. The narrative is viewed as an experience, not the true identity. This understanding provides better insight and allows for the reshaping of life stories. In narrative therapy, distancing from trauma occurs without avoiding emotional distress. The focus is on externalizing the experience rather than internalizing it to prevent emotions from getting stuck in the body.

Narrative therapy has the power to manage the following mental health problems:

- Depression
- Anxiety
- Post Traumatic Stress Disorder (PTSD)
- Complex grief
- Complex trauma
- Acute trauma
- Attachment issues

Narrative therapy is a powerful tool for healing after trauma. It encourages individuals to craft a narrative that promotes healing rather than perpetuating destructive patterns. By carefully selecting words to recount their traumatic experiences on paper, individuals can reframe their stories through a lens of healing and resilience. Research supports the effectiveness of narrative therapy for trauma survivors, with studies indicating its potential for fostering post-traumatic growth. This therapeutic approach empowers individuals to transform their narratives and embark on a journey toward healing and personal development.

The Impact of Narrative Therapy

In the process of telling your story, it is critical to revisit memories that caused you to live with trauma, which can be painful and emotionally distressing. You may prefer not to talk about your trauma and avoid topics related to your story. And who wouldn't?

Nevertheless, studies have indicated that suppressing trauma can increase intrusive thoughts about the traumatic incident. Often, the fear of facing the pain can be more intense than just facing it head-on. I like to think of it as the hero's journey. The hero can spend her life hiding from the dragon or facing it bravely. The hero often finds the dragon is a source of love and kindness rather than a force to destroy.

Sharing your story is a personal decision, so consider sharing with someone you trust and feel secure enough to be vulnerable. Find someone who can be nonjudgmental, compassionate, and empathic to provide an environment to accurately recount your story without giving a diluted version. Narratives help make sense of your experience and declutter your mind. Telling your traumatic story can provide relief in the following ways:

- Let go of the shame and attachment.
- Eliminate distorted beliefs.
- Lessen triggers by the memories.
- Feel empowered to heal.
- Tell an organized story.
- Understand and make sense of your experience.

Apart from the benefits of sharing your story, the narrative you shape influences personal development and identity. Your worldview, beliefs, expectations for treatment, the relationships you cultivate, and the boundaries you establish are molded by the way you communicate with yourself and others. Your narrative holds significant sway over your self-perception. The story you constructed may not accurately align or contribute to overall well-being. Overidentification of your narrative can lead to destructive behaviors. At the same time, under-identification may prompt you to conceal aspects of yourself, hindering the expression of authenticity.

The sweet spot is acknowledging your current narrative without having it define you. Understanding your current narrative and its influence on your life empowers you to initiate changes for a fresh start in retelling your story and recovering from trauma. Failing to grasp your narrative or know your life story allows it to drive your decisions unconsciously. No one wants the trauma "driving the bus." Left unchecked, this reactive response to trauma gradually infiltrates your sense of self and gains power over your identity.

Narrative therapy allows you to hold space for all the emotions that arise, giving full attention and acceptance to whatever is present. Once fully acknowledged, there is room to take a step back and gain perspective and distance from the trauma. Acceptance is where the healing transformation occurs. When you sit to write your story once again, you will likely notice a shift from the destructive and inaccurate details of your original story toward a stronger sense of self and a healthier identity in this revised story.

Identifying The Start of Your Story

As you write your story, sometimes it's hard to know where to start. If you have a story burning to come out, go ahead and start writing that down. If you need help figuring out where to start reflection on your life story, use the checklist provided as a guideline to help identify traumatic experiences in your life story.

Have you -

- Experienced physical, emotional, or sexual abuse?
- Undergone financial, emotional, or physical neglect during childhood?
- Been diagnosed with a life-threatening or chronic illness?
- Experienced unexpected hospitalization?
- Sustained injuries while playing a sport or working?
- Been involved in an accident?
- Gone through a divorce?
- Witnessed your parents' divorce?
- Experienced or witnessed domestic violence?
- Lost a loved one?
- Grown up in a house with someone who was diagnosed with a mental disorder?
- Faced homelessness at any stage of life?
- Experienced a natural disaster?
- Raised in a household classified as having a low economic status?
- Been bullied at school, church, or work?
- Encountered discrimination against you?
- Lived with family members who engaged in substance abuse?

Trauma does not always need to be negative. Trauma reactions can also be experienced during happy moments, like childbirth. Suppose you do not relate to any of the traumatic experiences given above. In that case, it may be because you cannot recall any traumatic event. However, a close family member has mentioned it before. Hearing stories can also result in a trauma response.

Look at the checklist below and check the behaviors that match your life story. Let's get to the bottom of what happened to you.

- Experienced a fear of separation from your parents as a toddler.
- Recall having nightmares.
- Encountered weight problems or a poor diet.
- Faces difficulty concentrating.
- Struggles with falling asleep at night.
- Engaged in self-harming activities.
- Recalls feelings of depression and loneliness.
- Relied on drugs or alcohol as an escape.
- Became sexually active at a young age.
- Disconnected from reality, emotions, or the body.
- Characterized as a highly anxious person.
- Consistently feels tired.
- Becomes easily emotional when watching a movie or listening to a song.
- Displays quick anger and irritation with others.
- Frequently jumps to conclusions.
- Regularly recalls disturbing moments from a past traumatic event.
- Shows up differently in relationships.
- Adopts workaholic tendencies and refuses downtime on off days.
- Struggles to connect with the experiences of others.
- Believes that understanding is lacking in others.
- Maintains extreme caution regarding personal safety.
- Avoids engaging in small talk.
- Lacks interest in previously loved activities.

Narrative Therapy Exercise

Journaling your story is one of the therapeutic techniques used in narrative therapy. Writing a personal narrative may be simple and easy for some who have a story they are burning to tell. However, words might take time to come.

Here is a tip before you start: Begin with whatever comes up first, or start with the events leading up to the traumatic event, whichever feels right. Write your story to immerse an imaginary reader in your personal experiences, detailing everything you recall. The detail would allow them to perceive, sense, and undergo precisely your experience.

To help you get started, use these journal prompts:

- The best, strangest, and worst thing that ever happened to me
- The moment my life changed forever
- An experience that made me who I am today
- An unresolved problem in my life
- An event, object, or person that triggers me
- A false belief I cling to
- A childhood memory

Note that journaling about your trauma may be triggering or cause emotional distress. Remind yourself that sharing your story is a personal choice and that this should be done at your own pace. Take a break and give yourself grace when needed. If you are not ready to face this challenge, simply set this book down, engage in your favorite healthy self-soothing technique, and sleep on it. Remember, you are the hero of your own story. How and when will you show up for your story?

Begin by authentically expressing your story using all the words and emotions that surface in the present moment. This initial draft is a raw and unfiltered expression of your experiences and feelings. Rewriting and reframing your narrative will come later, allowing you to explore and process your story more intentionally and healingly. By first allowing yourself to articulate your thoughts and emotions freely, you create a foundation for deeper reflection and transformation as you navigate your healing journey.

INTERACTIVE ELEMENT

Grab a pen and write your life story to start your journaling exercise. You'll find the Chapter 2 prompts in the Free Interactive Elements Workbook to begin journaling your life story. Then, you will be ready to move on to the next step!

The Next Step

Now that you have written your narrative, you can start the process of changing it. I will guide you through this process throughout the following several chapters. So, no need to start editing your first draft today. Settle in and keep reading. Rewriting a life story encourages you to introspect and begin a process of self-discovery. Your upgraded story will practically write itself once you complete the steps this book discusses.

It involves asking yourself:

- What story have I been telling myself and others?
- Are there any recurring events?
- Is the story I am telling authentic, positive, and meaningful?

- What beliefs should I keep, and which do I let go?
- Which parts of my story serve my higher self, and which should I release?

Rewriting your narrative means taking control and creating a new story that promotes your well-being. When you change your story, you don't change the facts. You will reframe it to help you tell a more empowering story to yourself. Rewriting your story is about moving forward and releasing the narrative holding you back. Creating a new life story creates a meaningful and fulfilling life.

When you rewrite your story, avoid creating a delusional tale about the bad things that happened in your life. Instead of being in denial or painting yourself a picture that your life has been beautiful and happy since the day you were born, be authentic by embracing the mistakes and bad things that occurred throughout your life.

Some books and websites offer guidance on narrative therapy and storytelling for healing.

- *"Retelling the Stories of Our Lives: Everyday Narrative Therapy to Draw Inspiration and Transform Experience,"* by David Denborough.
- https://nathanbweller.com/tree-life-simple-exercise-reclaiming-identity-direction-life-story/

○ Scan this QR Code to access the link above.

SEGUE

When you have a clearer understanding of your trauma narrative, you are ready to move on to explore how to rebuild your strength in Chapter 3. To experience the most impactful results from this book, sit with these first two chapters and complete your initial journal writing before moving to the next step. This approach provides a foundation for the work ahead and grounds you wherever you are on your healing journey.

3

KNOCKED DOWN BUT NOT OUT

Success consists of getting up just one more time than you fall.

— OLIVER GOLDSMITH

Trauma has a strong force that will make you feel extremely weak. It makes you want to keep lying on the ground after being knocked down. Life might have hit you with one traumatizing event after another, but to successfully heal from it, you have to get back up every single time. It's a mindset you cultivate that will push you to rise after you fall.

Here is the inspiring story of Tiffany Holt, a resilient woman who endured trauma:

When Tiffany Holt reflects on her tumultuous childhood, she remembers a life filled with instability and challenges. When she was just five years old, her father came out of prison after five years, leading to a life of moving from place to place. Tiffany navigated through more than ten different elementary schools and saw the repercussions of her father's drinking problems, which often left the family in difficult situations.

"My dad would drink so much that he wouldn't go to work," Tiffany recounts. "We moved frequently; sometimes, six of us squeezed into a one-bedroom apartment." The constant upheaval took a toll on Tiffany's sense of security, prompting questions about love and belonging. "I often wondered if I was loved or hated," she reflects.

The only solace came from her hardworking mother, a figure of strength amid the chaos. "The only person who ever told me they loved me was my mom," Tiffany adds, her voice resonating with the echoes of a challenging past.

As Tiffany navigated adolescence, the challenges intensified. At 15, she returned from summer break to discover that her father had sold all their belongings and the trailer they called home. Forced to move in with her grandmother, the family endured cramped quarters, sharing a one-bedroom apartment. The financial strain led Tiffany to take on a job, a responsibility she shouldered to secure essential school supplies and new shoes.

"My mom could barely pay the rent, and my dad was practically useless," Tiffany recounts, painting a stark picture of a dysfunctional household where her father's alcohol-fueled aggression left a lasting impact. "He often took his frustrations out on my mom or my brothers. In 9th grade, I came home to pools of blood on the floor. My dad had tried to take his own life."

Tiffany found refuge in school—a sanctuary she regarded as her "safe haven." "School was my refuge, a place where I felt safe," she acknowledges, shedding light on the behavior of students experiencing trauma. Research indicates that some seemingly well-behaved students may be in a state of fear and survival.

Fortunately, Tiffany had a beacon of support in her life. At 16, she faced the prospect of dropping out of school to escape her tumultuous home life. However, recognizing her potential, her youth pastor and his wife intervened. They extended an invitation for Tiffany to move in with them, enabling her to continue her education away from the shadows of her father's alcoholism and her mother's struggles.

This pivotal intervention changed Tiffany's life. Celebrating her 16th birthday with a party, gifts, and a sense of belonging, she experienced a stark contrast to the hardships of her earlier years. "I broke the cycle, and I know that if other kids had that one person in their life, they too could break their cycles and be resilient," Tiffany asserts, underscoring the transformative power of mentorship and support.

As Tiffany set out to become an educator, she brought with her the wisdom gained from her turbulent past. "We are deeply invested in the well-being of our students. We aim to see them thrive, recognizing that meeting their basic needs is fundamental to fulfilling their academic potential."

Tiffany's message reminds us that intervention and support, though belated in her life, can have a profound impact. "I was a victim of trauma—neglect, abuse, and household dysfunction," she shares. Tiffany emphasizes the importance of early detection and support. "If someone had noticed I was going through trauma at a younger age, maybe I wouldn't have been exposed to as much."

Today, Tiffany leverages her experience to inspire others and advocate for student's safety and success. By building strong connections with her students and their families, Tiffany strives to provide the support and detection needed to break the chains of adversity and pave the way for resilient futures.

This chapter focuses on the role of resilience in healing from trauma and how self-worth and cultivating positivity build resilience.

THE ROLE OF RESILIENCE IN HEALING FROM TRAUMA

Tiffany Holt has shown you the role resiliency plays in coping with trauma. Despite her harsh and destructive environment, she rose above her circumstances. Tiffany could have easily chosen a path that led her astray—the same path her father took. Tiffany was resilient and more robust than the trauma she endured. According to research, the factors that promote resilience include positive temperament, sociability, optimism, and control of one's life. Tiffany Holt seems to have most of these qualities.

After a traumatic event, it is expected to experience a temporary decrease in your daily functioning. Your support network also plays a role in your ability to be resilient when coping with trauma. Many people refrain from socializing and instead choose to isolate. You may form distrust and other negative beliefs about your friends and family. You would rather spend days alone than with people you predict will stab you in the back. Pushing people away and isolating yourself adds to poorly recovering from trauma. Tiffany's safe space was her school, and her support system consisted of her youth pastor and his wife. These are factors that contributed to her resilience.

The role of resilience is to help you get up when trauma knocks you down. Resilience is the factor that holds a hand out for you and allows you to stand up after you have fallen. Resilience is an attitude and a mindset that acts as a protective layer when something traumatic happens. Trauma may have affected you deeply, but your resilience will motivate you to keep going even in adverse times.

PRACTICAL RESILIENCE STRATEGIES

Resilience is essential since you cannot control how your life will unfold; you can only choose how you deal with it. Build your resilience to cope during adverse times with these three practical strategies:

Keep Going No Matter What

After trauma, your mind may be working against you rather than with you. You will try to avoid facing the problems and sweep them under the rug. You try anything to escape the harsh reality of what happened. Trauma can leave you feeling unmotivated and lead to a sedentary lifestyle. Trauma has a way of chipping away your enthusiasm, hope, and excitement.

How do you flip the script for your brain? Staying motivated will keep you going, no matter your circumstances. Boosting your energy levels and motivation involves taking action. Simply making your bed and cleaning your room can build momentum for the day ahead.

Here are seven tips to enhance motivation:

- **Determine your goals:** How will you feel when you achieve the goals you have identified? Sit with that feeling for a while.
- **Boost your endorphins:** Engage in any activity that increases your happy hormones, such as exercising for 30

minutes daily, exposing yourself to sunshine, spending time with those you love, and practicing gratitude.

- **Create a consistent routine:** A solid routine provides structure and stability. It also reduces your "cognitive load, " giving you more brain power to tackle other things.
- **Identify your "why":** You may feel ashamed, fearful, have a depressive episode, or be lethargic. Then, ask yourself why you want to keep going. Finding the answer to your "why" will increase your enthusiasm and motivation.
- **Find people who motivate you:** Identify a mentor who inspires you to keep going. Find that one person in your life who energizes you. This person could be someone who has gone through the same experiences or someone who supports and motivates you. Remember, the person or people you choose as mentors don't have to be experts. Realizing that there are people who have your back during tough times will keep you going in the right direction.
- **Do not compare yourself to anyone:** You can be motivated by the success of others, but avoid comparing yourself to them. Your only competition is yourself! Be encouraged to keep going and to do better than you were yesterday. Strive to be better every day.
- **Practice self-care:** Self-care promotes mental and physical energy, helping you stay motivated while healing from trauma. Reward yourself and celebrate your progress as you continue your healing journey.

Give yourself grace on days when you feel unmotivated. You have the tools to get back on track. NEVER wait for your motivation to return! Take action to increase your motivation.

Increase Your Self-Worth

What does knowing your value mean to you? Why is it essential to build resiliency? *Self-worth is defined as how you evaluate yourself: Am I capable, valuable, and deserving of respect from others?* Self-worth comes down to how you feel about yourself, your perspective of who you are, how you talk about yourself, and what you believe you deserve.

As a woman, whether you're excelling in your career, fulfilling the role of wife, or nurturing as a mother, it's vital to embrace and honor your true self. You may base your self-worth on the viewpoints of others. The truth is you define your self-worth. Trauma distorts your self-worth and creates destructive beliefs that you do not deserve to receive love or to have good things happen to you. When you are impacted by trauma, you tend to believe the things others say about you because your sense of self has been shattered. You lack confidence and strength, which makes you internalize and accept the opinions others have formed about you.

Test your level of self-worth with the questions below:

- Do you respect and value yourself?
- How do you usually describe yourself to others?
- Is your inner dialogue negative or positive?
- Do you feel worthy of receiving love and respect from others?

Introspection to find the answers to the above questions will help you define your low, normal, or high self-worth. By increasing your self-worth, you become a more confident woman who's able to separate the opinions of others from how you choose to define yourself. If you have high self-worth, you will have the confidence to experience stressful moments and have the ability to cope with anything that crosses your path. External events will not define you. You will have the confidence to pursue your goals and believe you will be healed no matter what.

Here are some strategies to increase your self-worth:

- Engage in activities that align with your passion and strengths.
- Challenge yourself to improve your overall being.
- Confront flawed thought patterns to change negative beliefs.
- Practice self-acceptance to recognize your worth.
- Do introspection to increase self-understanding.
- Show yourself love and compassion to believe you are worthy of good things.
- Set small, achievable goals, and reach them.

High self-worth is essential to resilience and managing stressful life events. It will benefit you when coping with the adverse effects of trauma and provide you with a positive, hopeful, and self-assured mindset.

Cultivate Positivity

Realistic optimism offers a shield for adverse events that occur in your life. It allows you to acknowledge the situation as alarming, threatening, or traumatizing. Your mindset will tell you, *Yes, life is hard right now, but you got this. You can handle this situation*!

Realistic optimism allows you to perceive situations as they are without altering your self-perception. Your inner voice remains encouraging and compassionate rather than critical.

Realistic optimism is a regulation tool that helps you process and get through challenging times. Suppose you naturally gravitate toward negative thinking patterns during hard times. In that case, you can still learn to rewire your brain by nurturing positivity with the following strategies:

- **Practice gratitude regularly** and integrate thankfulness into your lifestyle. For instance, determine at least five things you are thankful for each morning or night.
- **Find meaning** by pursuing the activities that make you happy and fulfilled. Follow your dreams and passions, and make a difference for others.
- **Be in the moment** as often as you can. If you are taken back to the past or worrying about the future, allow yourself to feel the emotion, then let it go.
- **Focus on what is good, useful, and helpful,** and give less attention to the aspects of life that drain your energy, make you feel unworthy, and generate negative thoughts.

Next is the story of Katharine, who showed true resilience throughout her life.

In her early 40s, Katharine embarked on a journey of self-reflection, unveiling a life marred by trauma that began in her tumultuous childhood. Recounting the harsh treatment from her parents, she shared, "My dad beat me with his belt for minimal altercations like popcorn kernels on the floor," shedding light on the harsh realities she faced.

As a member of the Distributive Education Clubs of America (DECA) in high school, Katharine faced further challenges when her father punished her for crying when she couldn't secure a ride for her DECA Program work permit. This punishment escalated to physical abuse, adding another layer to her already complex narrative.

"At age 15, I attended school between 7:00 and 11:30 AM and began working three jobs after school, but still kept my grades up. I'd get home around 11:00 PM and do homework and laundry," Katharine revealed, showcasing her resilience despite the adversity. However, her parents asked her to move out after her junior year, leading her to find an apartment near her school without informing anyone.

Katharine's life took a dark turn during a visit from two police officers responding to complaints of prowlers; she experienced sexual assault and threats that persisted for months. Despite the ongoing abuse, she chose to remain silent about the ordeal.

It became clear during Katharine's senior year that her parents did not intend to help her pursue a college education as promised. Meeting David, a TV personality, at the Dallas airport gave Katharine an escape, leading her to Los Angeles after high school. Uncomfortable in the entertainment scene, she eventually left the job due to financial struggles, returning to Alabama.

In Alabama, Katharine lived with a girlfriend and owned a car she had bought herself. She was hospitalized for extreme dehydration due to tonsilitis when her parents forged her name and sold her car. Katharine persevered and secured a job in a law office.

A car accident during a trip with a friend exacerbated her childhood back injuries, with five spine surgeries beginning at age 15. Katharine's life took a positive turn when she met Leighton, who had relocated to Alabama from Florida. During her post-surgery recovery, he visited daily for four weeks. Upon recovery, she had a job waiting for her. The couple married, relocated to Mississippi, started a family, and attended church. They aimed for a big family and raised their children in the Christian faith. Adapting from her upbringing, Katharine learned proper discipline methods and began homeschooling their five children.

At 38, Katharine faced new challenges with health issues, including myalgic encephalomyelitis/chronic fatigue syndrome (ME/CFS). She had begun to lose feeling in her legs. The rods in her back had been replaced after the car accident, but now Katharine needed surgery again. She endured pain that she had never felt before and recovered at home with a wheelchair. The ME/CFS diagnosis prompted Katharine and her husband to find a Christian school, as she could no longer homeschool.

The trauma continued to haunt Katharine's life, from her parents' abusive actions to financial strains and health battles. Opening up to a counselor, she unraveled her traumatic past, revealing a childhood marked by negligent caregiving responsibilities due to her mother's mental health struggles and her father's neglect.

The recent years have brought more trials, including rebuilding their home after a tornado and ongoing family discord. Katharine faced a series of health crises, including a tractor-trailer accident, a misdiagnosis of blood cancer, and a breast cancer diagnosis, leading to a mastectomy, surgical errors, and ongoing medical treatments that caused weight gain and liver damage.

In December 2023, Katharine found herself in the hospital, suffering from dehydration as a result of a virus. The situation escalated when she collapsed in the bathroom, resulting in a broken leg. "I'm constantly bracing myself for the next unfortunate event," she admits. Katharine's health challenges extend beyond this incident. She struggles with adrenal fatigue, a condition that causes her adrenal gland to produce insufficient cortisol levels due to a lifetime of being in a fight-or-flight state. Additionally, she grapples with Post-Traumatic Stress Disorder (PTSD). Even innocuous actions, like the sound of her husband removing his belt, can trigger her despite knowing he poses no threat.

Despite it all, Katharine copes by finding humor in her stories, telling them lightens the heaviness she carries. "I can't be the grandma I want to be, but I can enjoy life for myself and those I love," she shared, emphasizing the importance of finding joy amid adversity. Katharine's husband has been her caretaker for 24 years, and together, they find solace in their Christian faith, supported by the kindness of their 12 grandchildren, with one more on the way. Through it all, Katharine searches for purpose, embracing the love surrounding her in the face of life's relentless challenges.

INTERACTIVE ELEMENT

The Build Your Resilience worksheet is in the Free Interactive Elements Workbook for Chapter 3.

SEGUE

Enhanced resilience prepares you to build on your foundations in Chapter 4.

THE REBUILD BEGINS

Trauma is a fact of life. It does not, however, have to be a life sentence.

— PETER A. LEVINE

The quote suggests that although you have endured trauma at some point in your life, the impact of it doesn't have to be permanent. Yes, it happened, but you determine if it's a life sentence or just a chapter in your life. You can find light at the end of the tunnel and emerge stronger from this season of your life.

Below is the story of Jamie, who transforms her life after trauma and leaves you with some words of wisdom (Women Against Abuse, n.d.):

Jamie's transformative journey unfolds as she shares, "For six and a half years, I endured extreme emotional, mental, physical, and even financial abuse at the hands of my ex-partner." She recalls Peter

Levine's insightful message as she reflects, "Yes, it happened, but you determine if it's a life sentence or just a chapter in your life."

"I was completely isolated, broken, and defeated. It wasn't only my life that was in jeopardy, but also that of my daughter." In her attempt to conceal the harsh reality, she adeptly masked her pain with a brave facade, all while suffering immensely. "I was afraid to tell anyone what was happening in my home, afraid no one would believe me, especially since we both had high-profile roles in the martial arts community."

Jamie describes the gravity of her situation, "I was alone, without anyone to turn to, with my family in another state and no friends." She confronts the daunting decision of whether to leave and live or stay and succumb to the consequences. "He controlled my physical appearance, where I went, who I spoke to, and even my thoughts! He broke my spirit down to the point that I gave up my dreams and aspirations."

Detailing the harrowing experience of homelessness, Jamie shares, "My daughter and I walked the streets with a bag of clothes and a few of her favorite toys stacked on the stroller." The turning point occurred when she bravely escaped an attack, seeking refuge at a police station. However, her worst fear materializes as her ex-partner falsely claims abuse, resulting in her arrest.

Jamie discovered and tirelessly utilized the resources of Women Against Abuse. "I learned I had to relentlessly pursue safety, shelter, and support. I refused to take 'no' for an answer." Eventually, Jamie's perseverance paid off as she found solace with a supportive housing organization, Safe Haven, shedding the weight of years of abuse.

"In a single moment, years and years of abuse fell off my shoulders, and I felt a weight had lifted, which then gave birth to a new outlook, "Jamie stated. The narrative captures her journey of forgiveness, self-discovery, and empowerment. "I was NOT a victim. I had survived. At that moment, I took responsibility for my life and my daughter's."

Jamie describes her triumphant evolution," I went from being homeless, broken, insecure, and defeated to a driven and confident advocate, coach, speaker, and influencer. My voice has been heard on every platform, from Seventeen Magazine to The University of Pennsylvania to the State Capitol. I even went on to win my first World Title!"

This chapter guides you to take the first steps toward rebuilding your life after trauma. You will learn the importance of setting intentions and goals for your healing journey.

POST-TRAUMATIC GROWTH

This book can provide a guiding light for your inner journey and processing. Do you consider yourself more of an introvert or extrovert? Are you more open and transparent or deep and internal?

Studies show that if you possess the traits of openness and extraversion, you are more likely to experience post-traumatic growth. Openness lets you be transparent about new ideas, beliefs, and lessons learned from an experience. You will be accessible and not stuck in a thinking pattern that keeps you stagnant. Extraversion refers to focusing on gratification obtained from outside the self. If you consider yourself an extravert, you may allow new concepts into your life and accept help from people and belief systems that may not have been part of your life before.

Being open means letting go of wanting to control every situation and accepting external help and strategies that differ from your norm. These traits of extroverts naturally make you a person who gravitates toward others and seeks active ways to deal with your trauma. For example, you reach out to your support system when you hit rock bottom.

Some people may take a longer and deeper approach to PTG. While this may initially appear as a disadvantage, the deep internal reflection beneath the surface unveils a rich inner narrative that evolves with each experience. If this is you, your inner world acts as a shield against external pressures, enabling you to shape a deeply meaningful personal narrative far more meaningful than any external validation. External forces are less impactful to introverts, so you must consciously choose to alter your story from within.

It's understandable if you don't naturally possess the traits of openness and extraversion; it doesn't mean you're at a disadvantage when it comes to experiencing post-traumatic growth. A compassionate mental health professional can adopt a post-traumatic growth perspective in therapy, emphasizing the potential for growth and positive transformation. The therapist may wait until you reach a point in your healing process where you begin to show signs of positivity regarding the traumatic event.

Each individual navigates trauma uniquely, and my intent is that this book ignites inspiration and introspection, empowering you to embrace your journey with pride. It is important to remember that each person copes and recovers differently. But taking action is the way to make progress.

EMOTIONAL RESILIENCE

Post-traumatic growth and emotional resilience are both concepts related to how individuals respond to and cope with adversity, but they differ in their focus and outcomes. Emotional resilience refers to adapting and returning from difficult situations, setbacks, or stress. It involves maintaining a sense of well-being and functioning in adversity. Individuals with high emotional resilience can effectively cope with challenges, manage stress, and maintain a positive outlook after recovering from a crisis or trauma by regulating emotions and effectively managing their response to stress triggers. Emotional resilience means you feel the emotional response, but it doesn't bring you spiraling down.

Resilience helps you navigate and cope with the traumatic event smoothly, without the necessity of adopting a new belief system to make sense of life after the trauma. PTG refers to positive psychological changes that can result from struggling with a highly challenging life crisis. It involves personal growth, improved relationships, greater appreciation for life, and a deeper sense of personal strength. Post-traumatic growth can lead to a greater understanding of resilience and well-being after experiencing adversity. Resilience enables you to withstand trauma without it destabilizing your world.

It is possible for a person also to experience post-traumatic growth even if she bounces back quickly from a traumatic event. The speed at which someone bounces back does not necessarily determine her ability to experience growth. Some may take more time to process their experiences and find meaning in them. It is important to remember that everyone's journey toward growth is unique, as no specific timeline or threshold exists for experiencing PTG.

If you are resilient, you handle stressful situations calmly, while being less resilient means you react with negative emotions. For example, Pam and Desiree both got fired effective immediately. Desiree was disappointed but communicated assertively and calmly, packed her belongings, and left the premises. On the other hand, Pam was angry and started swearing at everyone who looked at her while packing her belongings. We later found that Desiree got a new job within two months while Pam was still at home, battling with depression.

Emotional resilience kicks in during a stressful circumstance. It enables you to collect yourself and bring you back to emotional safety after you have experienced a threat. Emotional resilience gives you the confidence and motivation to go through difficult situations, knowing you will come out strong on the other side. It's your mind being self-compassionate and walking you through adverse times. You may realize you are in a dark place, but your resilience allows you to handle this moment, knowing it is a temporary phase. Just keep going. Look at emotional resilience as a trait that will enable trauma to bend you but not break you.

Below are essential components contributing to emotional resilience:

- **Physical Strength:** Cultivate a robust physical foundation to withstand life's challenges, promoting overall well-being.
- **High Energy Levels:** Maintain vitality and stamina, enabling you to navigate demanding situations with vigor and endurance.
- **Optimal Health:** Prioritize good health practices to fortify your body, mind, and spirit, forming a resilient base for emotional well-being.

- **Adaptability to Change:** Develop the capacity to adjust and thrive in the face of evolving circumstances, fostering resilience in dynamic environments.
- **Extended Concentration Span:** This will enhance your ability to focus for sustained periods, contributing to effective problem-solving and emotional stability.
- **Elevated Self-Esteem and Confidence:** Nurture positive self-perception and unwavering confidence, empowering you to confront challenges with self-assurance.
- **Heightened Self-Awareness:** Cultivate a deep understanding of your emotions and reactions, laying the groundwork for informed and adaptive responses.
- **Emotional Regulation Skills:** Learn to manage and regulate emotions, promoting emotional balance and resilience in adversity.
- **Strong Cognitive Skills:** Develop practical, comprehensive abilities to navigate complex situations, fostering adaptability and problem-solving capacity.
- **Cooperative Nature:** Cultivate a collaborative mindset, enabling you to engage positively with others and navigate challenges collectively.
- **Teamwork Proficiency:** Hone your collaborative skills, leveraging collective strengths for resilient problem-solving.
- **Effective Communication:** Develop assertive communication skills, promoting understanding and collaboration in various contexts.
- **Robust Interpersonal Connections:** Build and maintain strong connections with others, creating a support network crucial for emotional resilience.

If you identify areas where you may lack resilience, recognize that resilience is a skill that can be developed. The key to emotional resilience lies in managing the challenges and safeguarding your emotional well-being.

Five Pillars of Resilience

In our society, we often celebrate success—the big wins, the achievements, and the moments of glory. But what about the moments in between?

Resilience is the quiet strength that allows us to weather life's storms, bounce back from adversity, and emerge stronger than before. It empowers us to rebound from adversity and emerge with enhanced fortitude. It allows us to endure hardships, rebound, and arise even stronger.

Resilience involves more than just enduring life's challenges; it's about embracing and cherishing the ebbs and flows of life. Difficulties shouldn't just be endured but approached with curiosity, an open mind, and a touch of love.

Your mindset plays a crucial role in your resilience. A growth mindset, characterized by a belief in our ability to learn and grow, can empower you to face challenges with courage and determination. It's about reframing setbacks as opportunities for growth and as stepping stones on the path to success.

Resilience is a skill that can be learned. Numerous studies have shown that using simple tools to look at life from the bright side can profoundly improve your resilience. It helps increase well-being and opens us to more significant social connections, improved sleep patterns, enhanced memory, better listening skills, and even more robust immune systems. With such a fantastic range of benefits, it is clear that taking a few minutes each day to focus on the positives can be profoundly life-changing!

The **Five Pillars of Resilience** can help you redirect your thinking and see yourself and the world differently and in new ways.

1. Self-awareness is a fundamental stepping stone that allows us to adapt to our environment and circumstances. Resilience is a natural byproduct of self-awareness. Understanding the self gives us an idea of our inner strength, allowing us to face challenges and difficult situations with self-assurance. Understanding yourself also gives you a heightened awareness of how others view you—your attitude, reactions, and motivations allow you to communicate with those around you more effectively.

2. Mindfulness is a compelling practice that can help us build resilience and thrive in body, mind, and spirit. It encourages us to get out of our heads and into the present moment, acknowledging thoughts or feelings without judgment and learning to respond to challenges with thoughts rather than emotions.

A regular mindfulness practice allows us to stay fully engaged with our life experiences, even during challenging times, allowing more openness in approaching life at every moment with heightened perspective and appreciation. Perhaps it's noticing beautiful colors like the dark blue sky, soft green grass, or the bright stars in the night sky.

3. Self-care ensures you are in the best possible condition to face life's challenges. It means different things to everyone. It's about ensuring you are physically, emotionally, and spiritually well enough to be available for others. It's about recognizing when to rest and recharge and allowing yourself to do so without feeling guilty.

It's about setting boundaries and saying *no* when you feel the need. It's about nourishing your body with healthy food, regular exercise, and restful sleep. Self-care that nourishes your mental and spiritual health could mean seeking therapy or counseling, meditating, or praying. Taking some moments to pause and reflect throughout the day can boost your energy and confidence. It's about doing the things you enjoy that make you smile and fill your cup so you're ready to help others!

4. Positive Relationships are the people who support and care for us — and we care for them. We don't have to face life's challenges alone. A strong support system can provide the encouragement, guidance, and perspective we need to navigate difficult times. Whether it's friends, family, mentors, or peers, having a support system can make all the difference in our ability to overcome adversity.

Connection with others helps us feel healthier, happier, and more satisfied with our lives. Sharing our struggles and triumphs creates a sense of community and solidarity. We can conquer obstacles together to find strength, resilience, and hope. By investing in positive relationships, we open ourselves to the incredible benefits of a deep sense of community; in today's world, having these powerful connections is more important than ever!

5. Purpose gives us a clear understanding of who we are and how we fit into the world. Believing in something bigger than ourselves can help us develop a positive attitude and a growth mindset to make us more resilient. Purpose could relate to a strong faith, relationships with family and friends, or using our talents to serve others. Additionally, we can find purpose in advocating for issues that are important to us. We can live better lives by recognizing that our actions have far-reaching consequences. This knowledge helps boost motivation and resilience.

Resilience is about maintaining inner peace and joy amidst the chaos, cultivating a mindset of growth and possibility, and building a support system that lifts us when we fall. So, let us embrace the journey, face challenges with courage and determination, and find strength, resilience, and joy along the way.

With perseverance, we can find inspiration to cultivate resilience and embrace the journey, whatever it may bring. Remember, no matter how many times you fall, you have the strength within you to get back up and rise again.

STEP-BY-STEP PROCESS FOR HEALING AND GROWTH

Healing is not a walk in the park. It is mentally and emotionally challenging. Sometimes, it feels like you put in so much effort, but you just can't see the results. On other days, you may find yourself crying and screaming, while on certain days, you will thrive and recognize how your efforts have contributed to your growth. You will require motivation, self-compassion, and patience throughout this healing journey.

But how do you start your healing journey? You acknowledge what happened to you and its impact on you. You must start a healing journey with a plan. Understanding the stages of healing will aid you in effectively navigating your healing journey.

Now, let's look at an outline of a step-by-step process for emotional healing:

1. **Increasing self-awareness:** Recognize the traumatic event and acknowledge the emotional distress you are experiencing. This step is crucial as it brings awareness to the source of pain, setting the foundation for your healing journey.
2. **Starting to acknowledge:** Accept the pain and trauma as integral parts of your life. By recognizing a problem that requires attention, you take ownership of your healing process and commit to addressing it head-on.
3. **Allowing the feelings:** Permit yourself to experience and process all intense and negative emotions without judgment or avoidance. Allowing these feelings to surface and be acknowledged is a vital part of moving toward healing.
4. **Recognizing the impact:** Acknowledge how the trauma and pain have affected the different aspects of your internal and external world. By understanding the far-reaching implications of these experiences, you can begin to address and heal the wounds they have caused.
5. **Getting resources:** Involves identifying the support and resources required to aid you on your healing journey. The resources may involve seeking assistance from individuals or organizations or identifying tools to support and guidance as you navigate the healing process.
6. **Rebuilding self-worth:** Focus on rebuilding self-esteem and self-confidence while recognizing your inherent worth. This phase involves enhancing self-perception and understanding your value as an individual deserving of healing and growth.

7. **Learning self-mastery:** Emphasize the importance of self-control and mastery over your thoughts, emotions, and actions. Developing self-discipline and regulating responses is vital to fostering personal growth and resilience.

8. **Building emotional resilience:** Learn how to manage and regulate your emotions effectively. By nurturing emotional resilience, you equip yourself with the tools to navigate challenges, setbacks, and triggers with greater ease and composure.

PRACTICAL EXERCISES FOR YOUR HEALING JOURNEY

Setting intentions and goals are two aspects that will keep you motivated when you embark on your healing journey. Intentions and goals go hand in hand. Intentions align your heart and mind with a goal or purpose. For example, having a goal to increase self-love will touch your heart. You would then set intentions every morning that are congruent with your goal, such as practicing affirmations before leaving the house, enjoying a healthy breakfast, or prioritizing your needs over others.

Depending on your faith or spiritual beliefs, you can pray for God's help to meet your desires. When you set a goal, you may ask God to bring it into your life. However, when your heart and mind are aligned with your goals to achieve healing, you become a powerful force. Before setting intentions, you need to determine the goals you want to achieve. Use the following questions to help you set goals:

- What are your short-term and long-term objectives to achieve healing and growth?
- How would you describe the ideal life you aspire to lead?

- What resources do you require more of, and which should you reduce?
- What do you need to let go of to pursue lasting happiness?
- What tools are essential for your growth and achievement?

Grace, who survived a horrific car accident, says (After Trauma, n.d.):

"I set a new goal every day; it started with simply walking to the bathroom, then progressed to walking to the bathroom and back. These achievements evolved to tasks like walking to the end of my road with just a walking stick or doing my makeup with my left hand due to severe nerve damage in my right hand."

Everyone's healing goals will differ depending on the trauma they have experienced. Some healing goals involve changing your thinking style, growing in a positive direction, validating your truth, prioritizing your needs, establishing boundaries, and understanding that you will change as you heal.

You will discover how to establish intentions aligned with healing objectives. Follow these steps to create your intentions:

1. Begin by reflecting on your healing journey desires and articulating them in words.
2. Turn your words into a positive affirmation.
3. Consider revising the sentence if the words do not resonate with your heart and mind.

Intentions can be identified in the morning, before bed in preparation for the next day, or meditated on immediately. Write your intentions down when you choose to set them or say them out loud to yourself.

Calming Techniques to Practice

This section offers calming techniques to gain resilience during the healing process. Here is a list of ideas to calm yourself during adverse moments:

- **Mindfulness** is staying present in the moment and aware of the environment around you without judgment. It can be practiced while eating, walking, driving, or sitting still.
- **Breathwork** can be practiced by doing the 4-7-8 breathing exercises. Inhale for four seconds, hold your breath for seven seconds and then exhale for eight seconds. This method is one of many others. Find one that works best for you.
- **The Vagus nerve** can be stimulated in various ways. Begin by humming softly, gently touching your face, or splashing cold water. Another option is to engage in loud gargling with water or singing. Additionally, consider a foot massage using either a gentle or firm touch. Another effective method is to immerse your forehead, eyes, and at least two-thirds of both cheeks in cold water for a refreshing face immersion experience.
- **A grounding exercise** is called the 5-4-3-2-1 Technique. In it, you will name five things you see, four things you can touch, three things you can see, two things you can smell, and one thing you can taste.
- **Titration** helps slow down overwhelming emotions resulting from trauma by addressing them gradually. Focus on reducing the intensity of emotions and physical sensations. Work on one emotion at a time, pausing to listen and create space for each feeling. Prioritize the body's signals by giving them attention and time. This

approach helps manage emotions and bodily responses effectively.

- **Pendulation** oscillates your attention between the two areas of your body to build the capacity to handle negativity. You begin by choosing an area of your body that feels tense and holding your attention on it for a few minutes. Then, find a location in the body that feels calm or neutral. Tune into that part of your body and give it your full attention. Move back and forth between those areas to feel the difference consciously.
- **Empathy** shows gentle compassion by saying kind and soothing words to yourself.
- **Lean on your support network** by reaching out to a trusted friend or a contact in your social circle, or visit them to express and release your emotions.

INTERACTIVE ELEMENT

Chapter 4 of the Free Interactive Elements Workbook offers a Goal-Setting Worksheet. You will complete it and use it to track your progress.

SEGUE

With your goals in mind, you will dive into emotional healing and self-empowerment in Chapter 5.

EMOTIONAL FREEDOM

Whatever we plant in our subconscious mind and nourish with repetition and emotion will one day become a reality.

— EARL NIGHTINGALE

Feeding correct information to the subconscious mind increases your chances of achieving your goals. The subconscious mind controls most behaviors and dictates how you navigate life. We can control the subconscious mind through repetition and emotion. People who understand the power of the subconscious mind know the secrets to create a life that leads to emotional freedom.

Here is Jeanie's story about her therapy with a therapist named Cedric, who used emotional resolution as a therapeutic approach:

Jeanie's family endured an extended traumatic period lasting over five years, plunging them into a cycle of crises that ultimately led to

PTSD. Describing the emotional atmosphere during this time, Jeanie explains, "We were living in an emotional environment of panic, anxiety, fear, rage—all the emotions that developed as toxic defense mechanisms throughout the years of trauma." Unfortunately, the severity of each family member's trauma resulted in triggering one another instead of fostering love and support during conflicts or stress.

In their quest for help, the family consulted with over a dozen therapists, doctors, and psychiatrists, seeking individual and family support. Despite some relief from therapy and medication, the process of revisiting conflicts and reliving trauma proved exhausting. It yielded poor results, especially for the youngest family member.

Fortunately, Jeanie discovered Emotional Resolution through a recommendation. Expressing the uniqueness of this approach, she notes, "The brilliant thing about this work is, unlike many types of therapy, there is no rumination about any trauma that happened in the past." The technique, centered on breaking the physiological response cycle for triggers or situations, proved easily understandable, even for children. Jeanie initially brought her youngest to Cedric due to ADHD and the challenges stemming from a tumultuous upbringing, specifically anxiety, impulse control, and emotional regulation. The immediate and effective results prompted the entire family to engage with Cedric.

Reflecting on the transformative work, Jeanie asserts, "The results were immediate and so effective that we all started seeing Cedric." Through Cedric's efforts, the family underwent a healing process, addressing triggers, moving beyond trauma, and reclaiming the ability to live thoroughly once more.

Emotional freedom is a feeling that frees you from the emotional burdens that come with the trauma you have been carrying. Emotions are part of being human, so escaping them will never happen. You may enjoy experiencing positive emotions, while negative ones strip away your ability to enjoy life.

Emotions can give you information about yourself that you might not know, such as what you are passionate about and what threatens your safety. You will never be free from all your emotions, but you can learn to manage the feelings that feel like a burden. In Chapter 4, you will explore strategies for emotional healing and learn how to free yourself from the grip of traumatic emotions.

THE IMPACT OF TRAUMA ON EMOTIONAL REGULATION

Instead of feeling your emotions and dealing with them at the moment, you may avoid or squash the feelings. On the day of the traumatic event, and while suffering from the aftermath, you might have told yourself, *I don't have time to deal with this. I have things to do.* Whether you distract yourself, minimize the emotional pain, engage in self-criticism, mask your emotions, or try to control and worry, you deny yourself from regulating your emotions and healing from trauma.

You might often choose to escape from your internal world when faced with vulnerability. Intense emotions bring uncomfortable sensations in the body. You run to anything that will alleviate those sensations, such as suddenly wanting to clean the kitchen, scrolling through social media, saying negative things to yourself, overeating, or excessive online shopping. By avoiding and squashing your emotions, you put yourself at risk for developing cardiovascular problems, and you increase your chances of developing cancer, depression, and anxiety. Sweeping your feelings under the rug may also cause issues within your social life, especially in your romantic relationships. Your bottled-up emotions can come to the surface in unexpected moments.

Consider trying a new approach to handling your emotions to avoid the consequences of suppressing, avoiding, and ignoring emotions. Challenge yourself to sit with your feelings. Note that you will be at your most vulnerable, and it will be uncomfortable at first. Instead of using your coping skills to protect you from the fear of being vulnerable, allow yourself to slow down and take it easy. You will benefit when you let yourself feel your emotions. Experiencing your emotions and vulnerability won't be easy, but it will be worth it.

By allowing your emotions to be present, you allow your nervous system to heal. Then, your body knows it is safe and no longer in danger. The body starts to recognize that the threat is gone, and you can now be compassionate and kind to yourself. Being present with your emotions makes life meaningful, helps you manage stress, enhances decision-making skills, promotes mental health and growth, and makes you more resilient.

Emotions as Messengers

Is it normal for you to minimize your emotions? If so, you may need help understanding the message your emotions want you to receive. If you disallow yourself from feeling a particular emotion, you will not see the true meaning of experiencing it. If you deny the emotion, you deny the message it's trying to send you. Emotions serve as messengers, conveying valuable insights about yourself and your surroundings. By acknowledging and understanding these emotions, you can respond to them effectively.

Negative emotions are healthy and human. As humans, we experience both positive and negative emotions. Let's say you are angry and view this emotion as wrong. You tell yourself, *I shouldn't be angry; I am just making a big deal out of nothing.* Your anger is trying to tell you something is wrong. Know that every emotion you feel is valid and worth acknowledging. Ignoring your feelings leads to an increased amount of emotional distress. Listen to your emotions, observe the action they want you to take, and then use that information to make your next move.

In the following table, you will learn the message each emotion wants to send you.

Emotion	Message
Anger	Protects you from a threat in your environment.
Sadness	Notifies you that you have lost something valuable.
Guilt	Directs you to correct your wrongdoings.
Hurt	Guides you in resolving the issue you're facing.
Anxiety	Prepares you for future situations or to manage your current problem.
Lost	Tells you to seek guidance for feeling adrift and unknowing.
Provoked	Indicates solid and unwelcome feelings that you need to address a harmful situation.
Apathetic	Signals disinterest that you are not connected to your emotions.
Helpless	Informs you to take control when you are unable to defend yourself.
Frustration	Indicates you need to try something new when you feel defeated.
Fear	Provides you the energy to protect yourself from harm.
Desperation	Specifies that something terrible is required when you feel anguish.
Burdened	Alerts you that you need external help.
Awkward	Connects you to the present moment when you feel ungraceful.
Discontent	Associates dissatisfaction with your unmet needs.

Disgust	Signifies strong disapproval to keep away from something.
Antsy	Vigilant impatience to resolve the problem.
Stubborn	Signals that you are closed off to receive new information.
Wary	Shows caution and watchfulness to act.
Ambivalent	Gestures with mixed feelings or contradictory ideas lead to uncertainty.

Each emotion has a message for you. Before disregarding your feelings, decipher the hidden message they are trying to send, then act on that underlying message. Unresolved trauma has a way of showing up in your emotional responses. You may respond in one of two ways: showing no emotion or feeling intense emotions. When something traumatic happens, you may experience an absence of feeling—emotional detachment. On the other hand, you might notice yourself getting angry more often or crying for no reason.

Trauma impacts your ability to regulate your emotions. If trauma occurred early in your life, you could have a problem regulating emotions. In contrast, a trauma in adulthood may only cause a short period where you will struggle to soothe or control your emotional responses.

Living with unresolved trauma can present significant challenges, manifesting in difficulties regulating intense emotions and coping with stress. The struggle to manage anger or anxiety within interpersonal relationships can result in irreparable harm. Furthermore, individuals may resort to unhealthy coping mechanisms in an attempt to regulate their emotions, creating a dangerous dilemma. Engaging in risky behaviors such as substance abuse, gambling, or compulsive actions exacerbate the already complex effects of trauma.

How to Manage Your Emotions

Not everyone who experiences trauma develops unhealthy coping skills to deal with the aftermath. Some people engage in healthy coping skills such as self-care, exercising, journaling, or leaning on their support system. However, in most cases, the coping strategies are only a distraction from the uncomfortable emotions experienced in the body, as the body cannot work through the trauma or emotions itself.

Here are four easy steps to process and manage your emotions:

1. **Take a minute** to pause and refrain from any activity. Stay mindful of the present moment and engage in a grounding exercise like counting to 20 or identifying five red objects in the room.
2. **Recognize the emotion** and determine its source. Validate your feelings by saying, "It's okay to feel the emotion." Next, identify the message your emotions are sending you.
3. **Plan to improve your emotional state** by focusing on changing it. Consider the sources of happiness in your life and strategize ways to access them.
4. **Take action** based on the decision made in step 3.

Step 3 could be the most challenging of all the steps mentioned. It encourages you to think of ways to improve your emotional state. Avoid engaging in destructive coping skills as a quick fix.

If you have trouble developing ideas for step 3, use the table below to make healthy choices.

Healthy Coping Skills	Unhealthy Coping Skills
Mood boosters (read, watch funny videos or a movie, clean, play with your pet)	Denial (refuse to accept reality, minimize or invalidate emotions)
Self-care (healthy eating, drinking water, sleeping appropriate hours, bathing, setting boundaries)	Withdrawal (disengagement from others, solitude, poor boundaries, insecurity, exploitation by others)
Process feelings (draw your emotions, allow yourself to cry, talk it out, punch a pillow)	Bullying (threaten, ridicule, hurt others, show dominance)
Problem-solving (list your strengths, brainstorm resolutions with someone)	Self-harm (engaging in risky behaviors that hurt you)
Performing acts of kindness (help out at a community center, do something nice for a stranger, walk a neighbor's dog)	Substance abuse (excessive drinking, using drugs)
Hobbies (write, draw, paint, dance, learn, play, cook, garden)	Negative habits that create self-sabotage (irrational behavior, negative self-talk, overeating, over-exercising, obsessive cleaning)
Relaxation exercises (break from social media, listen to music, practice yoga, deep breathing, meditate, play with Play-Doh, take a walk)	Hiding from the world, finding distractions (Sleeping too much or staying in bed to avoid action)
Support system (video call or text a friend/family member, sit with a trusted person, reach out to a therapist)	Settling for those who bring negativity to your life (gossip, criticism, or judgment)

Big emotions can be challenging to process. It's natural to want to run from those emotions as soon as you experience them. You no longer need to run.

Here are six strategies to follow when struggling to manage intense and uncomfortable emotions:

- **Recognize and decrease emotional triggers:** Identify the memories, people, places, objects, or situations that trigger an intense emotional response. This strategy suggests avoiding emotional triggers as much as possible. First, you must recognize and become curious about your triggers. Determine why this specific trigger holds power over you and seek ways to reduce its importance.
- **Tune into your body's sensations or physical symptoms:** When highly charged with emotions, identify the underlying factors that could add to your emotional state. The symptom impacts may include hunger, sleep deprivation, caffeine addiction, or anxiety.
- **Observe your thinking patterns:** When you are emotional, you may not think logically. You feel irrational when you don't know the whole story, so your mind fills in the blanks with negative assumptions. Instead, look at what your thoughts tell you and think of alternative answers.
- **Change inner dialogue to a positive one:** When emotions overwhelm you, your self-talk can turn negative. You may find your inner dialogue filled with self-criticism and doubt, leading you to believe these harmful thoughts. Make an effort to transform your self-talk into a positive conversation. Swap out a negative thought with a positive one to challenge irrational beliefs and alleviate negative emotions. Taking charge and being mindful of your self-talk during these moments is crucial.

- **Choose how to respond:** Avoid responding impulsively to questions, comments, or circumstances, as this ruins relationships and opportunities. When you recognize a negative emotion, tell yourself, *I choose how to respond to my feelings.* This affirmation will help you respond more effectively to situations that spike your feelings.

- **Actively seek positive experiences:** Humans tend to pay more attention to negative experiences than positive ones, which could lead to poor mental health. However, when you focus your attention on positive experiences, you improve your emotional response and well-being. Savor the joyful moments, and express gratitude for their presence in your life.

Dave Chan reached out for help from a therapist, and this is his feedback after finishing therapy (Emotional Resolution with Cedric Bertelli, n.d.):

Emotional Resolution (EmRes) has changed Dave's life. Because of its simple yet effective sensory evoking technique, Dave could awaken to his true self through his physical body and live in the present moment. Dave states, "Although challenging at first, my commitment to personal growth, coupled with the expert guidance and compassionate teachings from a specialist, along with the support of the Emotional Resolution community, has enabled me to address my past conditioning and embrace a significantly more fulfilling life."

Sounds impressive, right? A more fulfilling life, free from past conditioning, isn't just for the select few. It is accessible to *anyone* willing to put in the work using the strategies discussed in this book. *You* can do this too. Be brave, take a deep breath, and forge ahead.

THE POWER OF A THOUGHT

Thoughts occur only in your internal world. Nobody else can hear your thoughts, only you. Thoughts are personal and ultimately create an understanding of your internal and external world. You live in this world with billions of others, experiencing the same events but with countless interpretations.

Frequently, you likely grant your thoughts more power than they deserve. The problem occurs when you treat all your thoughts as facts that should be believed. For instance, you want to try a new hobby, but your thoughts keep saying, *I can't do it*. Eventually, you believe it, thus never engaging in the hobby. Jon Kabat-Zinn claims that "a thought is just a thought," nothing more (Perelman School of Medicine, n.d.). If only it were that simple.

Thoughts are powerful, and your healing depends on what you decide to do with an idea when it pops into your mind. More than 100 thoughts enter your mind daily, but the ones you entertain hold the most power over your emotions and behavior. The thought will disappear if you choose not to give it any energy. Treating your thoughts like the sound of a car passing by your window may be helpful. Notice it, see if it is a current threat, then let it go completely.

Recognize that a thought is not necessarily a fact or a truth. An idea becomes genuine with the attention and interest you put into it. Many factors, such as your mood, emotional state, and worldview, influence your thoughts. Consider the following scenarios and how you would react to the situation:

- You are frustrated that you've had a bad day at work. When you get home, your partner asks, "What's up with you?!"

- You are in a fantastic mood and just got a job promotion. When you get home, your partner asks, "What's up with you?!"

It's the same situation, but your reaction and thought pattern toward the question will differ depending on your mood. Thoughts and emotions share a profound relationship, as thoughts can determine your feelings. At the same time, emotions can also fuel specific thoughts. Your thoughts are always dependent on any number of factors. Therefore, you should take your thoughts with a grain of salt. Thoughts shouldn't be ignored; they should be allowed to exist without taking them too seriously by letting them leave peacefully.

To allow a thought just to be a thought, practice the following mindfulness exercise to observe your thoughts analytically (Perelman School of Medicine, n.d.):

1. **Focus your attention** on your breathing pattern until you feel a sense of calmness flush over you.
2. **Become aware of the thoughts** that arise while you focus on breathing in and out.
3. **Accept any thoughts** that arose in Step 2, whether negative or positive. Allow your thoughts to exist and avoid attaching any meaning to them.
4. **Reframe your thoughts** as they may be hyper-focused on correctly completing this exercise, and you may be telling yourself, *I am not doing it right; this exercise won't work.* Reframe the thought: *This is just an exercise.*
5. **Use metaphors** to allow a thought to be nothing but a thought. Consider thoughts as leaves gently drifting on a flowing river, envision them as clouds passing through the vast expanse of the sky, or liken them to a captivating

performance unfolding on a theater stage or a movie on television.

6. **Let your thoughts play out** without entertaining, judging, or meaning. Allow them to pass quietly through your mind.
7. **Recognize a thought** and consciously see how quickly a new one replaces it.
8. **Bring your attention** back to your breathing pattern.

With the above exercise, you increase your awareness and regain power by not letting your thoughts control your actions, inner dialogue, or internal world.

What are Cognitive Distortions?

Cognitive distortions are erroneous thought patterns that amplify your perception of a situation, leading to a negative outlook. By intensifying thoughts, these distortions convince the mind to adopt pessimistic beliefs about oneself and the world. Despite lacking a factual basis, these distortions are often perceived as truth. They are prevalent among individuals, with many having experienced them at some point. Consistent engagement in cognitive distortions can have a detrimental impact on your mental well-being, potentially leading to a downward spiral in your mental health. Recognizing and addressing these distortions is crucial for maintaining a healthier mindset and outlook.

To avoid falling prey to distorted thinking, try to identify the following examples of cognitive distortions in your thinking pattern:

- **Polarization:** A thinking pattern that only allows you to see two perspectives is polarization. You will believe there are only two ways to understand the situation. For example, you may think you are a failure after an idea or project failed. In your mind, there is only failure and success, no in-between.

- **Personalization:** With this type of thinking, you turn everything toward yourself. You may believe it's about you in any situation when it might not connect to you at all. For example, eavesdropping on the conversation of two nurses while lying in the hospital bed. One nurse says, "I'm so tired; I wish my shift could end." Your thoughts tell you, *It's my fault the nurse is so tired. I need to get healthier so that I can go home.*

- **Jumping to conclusions:** In this situation, you predict what you think another person has done or implied without concrete evidence. This conclusion is your brain filling in the gaps where it doesn't have all the information to complete a story. For example, you see a colleague whispering to another coworker and automatically assume they are talking about you behind your back without considering other possible reasons for their conversation. It's essential to pause and gather more information before making assumptions. Jumping to conclusions is based on a thought or a belief that constantly dwells in your mind.

- **Overgeneralization:** This distorted thought pattern creates a belief about yourself, others, or situations based on one event. For example, your best friend betrays you, making you believe all women are traitors.

- **Filtering:** This thought pattern results when you disregard the positives in a situation and only focus on the negatives. An example of filtering is finding out you have been diagnosed with cancer. Your mind tells you that you are going to lose this battle. Of course, this diagnosis is severe and needs immediate attention. But, be careful not to ignore the fact that many people have survived and been cured of cancer.

- **Should statements:** These fall under the distorted thoughts category as they make you dwell on what you think you or someone else should have done. For instance, after being in an accident and waking up in the hospital, you think about everything you *should* have done differently to avoid the accident.

- **Catastrophizing:** This distorted thinking is about the worst-case scenario, which increases anxiety and negative thoughts about a situation. For example, when your partner doesn't message you, "I'm on my way home," like he always does before leaving work, you become anxious at the thought of him being in an accident on his way home.

- **Control fallacy:** An individual may perceive themselves as either a victim of circumstances (externally controlled) or believe they hold responsibility for the emotions of those around them (internally controlled). You either think you are in control or have zero control over something. An example would be lashing out at your colleague for not being considerate in front of others. You later tell another colleague that you had no control over lashing out because you were very angry at the moment.

- **Blaming:** This self-explanatory thought pattern occurs when you place the responsibility for your actions on someone or something else. For instance, you tend to treat your partner in an ill manner. When he confronts you about it, you blame your behavior on your traumatic childhood.

- **Emotional reasoning:** This cognitive distortion creates a strong belief that your emotions are factual. You feel scared and anxious when a man wants to pursue a romantic relationship with you. You believe that because those emotions are present, a relationship with this guy will unfold exactly like your last one.

Cognitive distortions are sneaky, as you might have created a habit of engaging in one of the distorted thinking patterns without realizing that it leads to negativity. Now that you are aware of unconsciously slipping into distorted thinking patterns, you will learn how to change them to cultivate a happier life and enhance your well-being.

Change Your Thinking Pattern

Your thinking pattern may occasionally need to be corrected. Still, it depends on what you do after the thoughts enter your mind. Will you entertain it and start believing it, or just watch it pass by like clouds in the sky? Identifying faulty thought patterns is essential to moving closer to framing situations in a more accurate and positive light. Then, when you identify a cognitive distortion, you'll know how to detach, erase, and let go of it.

Develop mental health habits that foster a rational thinking style. Jumping to conclusions or being hyper-focused on the negatives of a situation only leads to increased levels of fear and anxiety, while being mindful and present will reduce your stress. When you feel less anxious, you can make better choices and respond more effectively to stressful situations.

Here are five tips to erase a cognitive distortion and change your thinking pattern:

- **Become mindful of your thinking pattern:** Spend more time thinking about your thoughts. What thought pattern do you see most often? If something causes stress or feelings of anxiety, question what your thoughts are trying to tell you and whether they are accurate.
- **Be aware of how you communicate your thoughts:** Consider how you articulate your inner thoughts to the external world. Refrain from using absolute terms like "always," "never," and "nothing" and opt for more precise language. For instance, rather than stating, "You never care about my feelings," express, "I felt disappointed that my feelings were not taken into account today."
- **Note how you view yourself and others:** Avoid labeling yourself and others by their behavior. Behavior in isolated events does not define a person. Let's say your daughter felt exhausted today and decided to have a lazy day. Instead of labeling her as lazy for taking one day off, just acknowledge that your daughter didn't do any work for that day.
- **Seek out the positive:** When faced with a stressful situation that usually causes your thoughts to spiral, try to identify at least two positive aspects.
- **Find evidence before turning a thought into a belief:** Talk to others to gain more information, find evidence to support your thought, and question it before committing.

Distorted Past Memories

Did you know that memories of the past can become distorted? Though your brain is powerful, it is sometimes unreliable. We never question our memories and experiences because we trust ourselves. Research has shown that false memories are real.

Here are four ways research explains how memories can become distorted:

- **Change bias** refers to the tendency of individuals to prefer the status quo or resist change, even when change may be beneficial or necessary. It also explains how an individual might exaggerate a past event due to the stress experienced working toward change.
- **Cryptomnesia** is a phenomenon in which people believe they have come up with a new idea, concept, or creation. In reality, they have unconsciously remembered or been influenced by a previous idea.
- **Egocentric bias** occurs when individuals rely too heavily on their perspectives and fail to consider the viewpoints of others.
- **Illusory correlation** explains that memories can become distorted by creating an incorrect connection between two separate events.

Distorted memories can range from remembering childhood events as different from how they happened to recalling traumatic events that might still impact you today. You must sit with a family member, childhood friend, sibling, or cousin who has been there throughout your life to help you ensure that your memories of specific events are real, not false.

INTERACTIVE ELEMENT

The Free Interactive Elements Workbook contains two activities for Chapter 5 to assess and correct your faulty thought patterns.

If you haven't yet downloaded the workbook, use the QR code.

SEGUE

With newfound emotional resilience, you will explore maintaining calm and control in Chapter 6.

LEAVE A REVIEW!

Did you realize that one in three women will experience some form of traumatic life event?

My mission is to make emotional well-being accessible to every woman. Everything I do stems from that mission; reaching every woman is how to accomplish it.

I hope you find this book helpful. **Please leave an honest review on Amazon if you agree the book will equip you with the acquired skills and tools to overcome your past trauma.**

Use this QR Code to access the review link and leave your review.

Note: Use your applicable country's Amazon site for those outside the USA.

If you feel good about helping a faceless reader, you are my kind of person. Welcome to the club. You're one of us. Your honest review will mean the world to them and me!

I'm cheering you on!

Terri Sterk

COOL, CALM, COLLECTED

Calmness is the cradle of power.

— JOSIAH GILBERT HOLLAND

Fighting back, being angry, ensuring you are always safe, jumping to conclusions, and always having a response are often perceived as standing in your power and control. The truth is quite the opposite. It is difficult to reason when you are fueled with emotions acting from survival mode. After you have cooled down, you may not recognize the person you were while charged with emotion. Acting out of character is not healthy and could have detrimental effects on relationships and your well-being. Trauma causes you to be in a constant state of survival without realizing it. You might snap at someone quickly, always in a rush and ready to attack. Being in survival mode drives you to be defensive, hypervigilant, sensitive, and overprotective.

Living in survival mode for years can make being calm and slowing down look and feel foreign. It might even cause discomfort at first. However, you can regain your power and self-control when relaxed, calm, and collected. Being calm when triggered is difficult, but it is possible. Bringing yourself to a quiet state of mind has many benefits, such as making better decisions, avoiding intense emotions, and soothing the nervous system.

Let's look at the testimonial of Francesca, who started using calming techniques to improve her well-being (Madly Calm, n.d.):

The benefits of a regular Calmination Practice soothed Francesca during a particularly turbulent time. Engaging in a calming exercise allows her to disconnect from the chaos of daily life, entering a state of simply being to embrace the tranquility found in the union of self and breath. Francesca notes the positive impact: "The more practice I do, the quicker I can switch off and relax." She humorously acknowledges that her body craves this practice, with improved sleep and a noticeable reduction in backaches.

Reflecting on the transformation, Francesca shares, "I am conscious of checking in and slowing my breathing when I am particularly stressed, which is immediately soothing and calming." Notably, the practice has alleviated physical tension, such as unclenching her teeth and jaw, resulting in a more relaxed facial demeanor. Confronting her habit of shallow breathing, she has learned to consistently breathe slowly using her diaphragm, improving overall happiness and inner peace.

Expressing the impact on her perspective, Francesca attests, "I see things more clearly, and I no longer stress over little inconsequential things." Others have noticed, commenting on the positive change in appearance and the newfound sense of relaxation. Francesca emphasizes the positive influence of Calmination Practice on her mental health. She affirms, "I don't wake up feeling overwhelmed and anxious. If I feel nervous or anxious, I revert to slow, deep breathing, which helps immediately."

Chapter 6 focuses on helping you achieve emotional balance and develop coping strategies to navigate challenging moments with composure.

EMOTIONAL TRIGGERS

Experiencing emotional turbulence is similar to facing stormy weather. Like in a storm, staying calm during the emotional upheaval is essential to maintain a sense of calmness.

Similarly, in times of trauma, you must keep yourself composed and care for your inner self despite the challenging external circumstances. When recovering from trauma, your internal world is hypersensitive to your external world. Therefore, it's common to find yourself emotionally dysregulated. You may notice that your emotional reactions last longer than usual; you struggle to control your emotions and find it hard to adjust to different settings.

Next is Debra's story:

The trauma of losing a child is an unimaginable pain that no parent should ever have to endure. Debra Flanigan knows this pain all too well. Her world was shattered when she lost her beloved daughter, Casey, to Fentanyl poisoning in April 2023. The devastating loss of her oldest child left Debra grappling with grief, guilt, and a profound sense of emptiness. Amid her despair, Debra missed numerous treatments for her metastatic breast cancer, allowing the disease to progress. Casey, who had graduated high school, had put her life on hold to care for her mother, leaving Debra feeling the weight of missed moments with her two other daughters and three grandchildren.

Despite the overwhelming sorrow that consumed her, Debra found the strength to turn her tragedy into a powerful message of hope and resilience. Initially unaware of the dangers of Fentanyl, Debra now channels her courage, compassion, and unwavering determination to raise awareness about the lethal risks associated with the drug. Her tireless fight for justice for Casey is a testament to the steadfast spirit of a mother's love, becoming a beacon of light for others who have experienced similar heartbreak.

Debra's emotional triggers surfaced during a recent scan to monitor her cancer progression. "I prayed for good results, but when it went dark, all I could see were images of Casey," she shared. Overwhelmed by memories, Debra squeezed the emergency ball to signal the technician for assistance. She was unable to finish the scan that day. "I need to complete the scan, but I haven't rescheduled yet," Debra stated.

Before mastering emotional regulation skills, it is crucial to identify your emotional triggers. An emotional trigger can be a memory, experience, or event that evokes a strong emotional response, regardless of your current mood. Mood plays a significant role in reacting to emotional triggers, as certain moods can amplify your emotional responses. Emotional triggers can provoke consistent reactions based on the event, whether you are happy or angry. Understanding and managing these triggers is essential for emotional well-being and growth.

Emotional triggers are personal and connected to a past event in your life. You will notice that the emotional reaction to a trigger is not aligned with reality. For example, your friend can get behind the wheel and drive off, but when you want to drive, getting in the driver's seat spikes your anxiety. This emotional trigger exists as a result of a traumatic event that happened in the past. When you are emotionally triggered, the trigger takes you right back to the traumatizing event. When an emotional trigger pops up, you may feel vulnerable, unsafe, excessively uncomfortable, and overwhelmed with the emotions that are experienced.

Can you identify your triggers? Would you add anything to this list of common emotional triggers?

- Unresolved trauma
- Disturbing memories
- Past fears
- Stressful environments
- Interpersonal conflict
- Loss and grief
- Sudden or planned change
- A scent, a specific sound, or a person

How do emotional triggers form? When you experience a traumatic event, the brain stores this information in a different folder, usually outside of the conscious memory, compared to storing other information you receive from your environment. The brain does this for future purposes. Remember, the brain's main objective is to protect you from danger. The brain records traumatic memories and puts them in the *danger folder.* As a result of the information stored in the danger folder, the brain reacts with a fight-or-flight response when faced with a trigger.

Identifying Emotional Triggers

Emotional triggers always catch you off guard and cause chaos in your internal world. So, how will you take control and quiet the chaos? You take control by befriending your triggers. Get to know your triggers so that when you meet unexpectedly, you are already friends with them. When you can identify your triggers, you reduce the intensity of the emotional distress. Learn how to identify your triggers with the following tips (Josefowitz, 2021; Raypole, 2020):

- **Listen carefully to what your body is trying to tell you:** When you are emotionally triggered, what is your body's reaction? Record your body's physical response, such as sweating, nausea, increased heart rate, or lightheadedness. In addition, observe what emotions and thoughts pop up in your mind when triggered. This information about yourself will help you better prepare when your triggers creep up on you.
- **Pause and distance yourself:** It's best not to respond immediately to an emotional trigger. Avoid creating more chaos in response to the trigger. Take a step back and identify the trigger. Ask yourself, What exactly made me feel triggered? Familiarize yourself with the trigger to know the facts about it. In some cases, knowing the facts about a trigger teaches your brain new information about a stimulus initially interpreted as a threat.
- **Recognize a pattern:** Your emotional reaction to a trigger is automatic and happens so fast that you might miss the moment that led you to it. Identifying what led you to the emotional trigger can help you understand why you sometimes respond irrationally to a situation. By recognizing a pattern, you can break the pattern and

alleviate the stress that comes with a trigger, as you will feel prepared and have the tools to self-soothe.

- **Follow the paper trail:** It is helpful to think back and find moments when you experienced a similar emotional reaction. Triggers take you back to a past event or specific time in your life when you have experienced the same feeling you are experiencing when faced with a trigger. Finding the root of a trigger aids you in gaining a better understanding of yourself and your emotional triggers.

When you are triggered, don't be hard on yourself. Take a deep breath and gather information about your trigger. Know that confronting your emotional triggers won't be easy, and automatically responding to them might be an easier option, but remember you are working toward healing from trauma and breaking cycles.

How to Deal With Emotional Triggers in the Moment

When you become so overwhelmed with emotion that you want the feeling taken away immediately, you resort to the most accessible coping skill, no matter how unhealthy it may be. For instance, imagine being hit with a traumatic memory while talking to a problematic colleague at work. By being compassionate and assertive, you want to eliminate your emotions when dealing with the work associate.

Everyone loves a quick fix when it comes to dealing with uncomfortable feelings. But are those quick fixes healthy and effective, or do they complicate your issue in the long run? It's time to let go of all toxic methods of temporarily relieving intense emotions. Letting go is how you can manage emotional triggers and calm down within five minutes.

Check out the complete list of Self-Soothing Techniques in Chapter 2 to feel more grounded, centered, and safe in the moment. Some self-soothing examples are slow deep breathing, meditation, self-massage, snuggling with a pet, and journaling.

If healthy self-soothing isn't enough, refer to the Calming Techniques in Chapter 4. These will help you find calmness and gain resilience during this healing and de-escalating process. Calming techniques include mindfulness, breathwork, vagus nerve stimulation, grounding, titration, pendulation, empathy, ASMR, and leaning on a support network.

Another option is to explore autonomous sensory meridian response (ASMR) videos. ASMR refers to the sensation of tingling, static-like, or goosebumps that arise from particular audio or visual stimuli. These sensations can travel from the head to the neck and sometimes down the spine or limbs. Those who encounter ASMR frequently describe experiencing sensations of relaxation, tranquility, enhanced sleep, and overall well-being.

HOW TO PROCESS EMOTIONAL TRIGGERS LATER

It's great to have tools to help you calm down within five minutes because it makes you feel prepared, but these are quick fixes. Techniques that help you calm down within minutes won't help heal your anxiety or remove your automatic emotional response. Working on changing your emotional reaction involves rewiring the brain by repetitively practicing one or more techniques listed here.

Create a Self-Care Plan

Taking care of yourself nurtures the mind, body, and spirit. Start by creating a routine rooted in calmness and slowing down your life. Learn to be someone who plans their day and only does what you have time to complete. Consider your emotional capacity and plan accordingly. Avoid pushing yourself over your limit by adding more tasks to your plate. Self-care is about taking tasks off your plate and ensuring you are at ease.

Ensure that your self-care plan includes meeting your physical, emotional, mental, spiritual, financial, professional, and social needs. Playing should also be an essential part of your self-care plan as it boosts your emotional state, makes your inner child happy, and enhances your mental health. Playing teaches the brain to think creatively and makes you feel free to enjoy life.

Exercise Regularly

Exercising releases heavy emotions from the body and boosts your happy hormones. This technique can count as an in-the-moment method and will rewire the brain. You don't have to get a gym membership to move your body for at least 30 minutes daily. You can feel the benefits of exercising right away. Exercising allows the mind to feel safe and free from life's burdens. It sends a message to the brain, "It's okay. You can relax and enjoy the moment."

No specific exercise regime is required. Just do what feels good in the moment. Do you need explosive movement? Lift heavy things or run stairs. Do you need calming and loving attention? Try yoga, stretching, or a slow and steady bike ride. The point of this move-ment is to support what your body needs emotionally.

Develop the Habit of Good Sleep Hygiene

A good night's rest is crucial for our emotional regulation. Insuffi-cient sleep can lead to feeling cranky and being easily emotionally triggered. Many people tend to overlook the importance of sleep in their lives. Sleep hygiene includes before-bedtime activities, your sleep environment, and a consistent routine. To improve your sleep hygiene, start by

- making the room dark and quiet,
- ensuring the room is at a comfortable temperature,
- eliminating screentime before bedtime,
- doing a relaxing activity before bed, like meditating, reading, or journaling,
- avoiding the news or other distractions,
- staying away from caffeine, heavy meals, and alcohol before bedtime,
- creating a consistent bedtime routine and time for bed.

When it's time to sleep, your mind usually wants to remind you of everything you should worry about. Therefore, find ways to calm and relax your mind and body before sleeping.

Fill Your Life With Humor

You feel happy and cheerful when you laugh. Isn't that a feeling we all long to find? Sometimes, it feels out of reach when we are down in the dumps or triggered. Making a conscious effort to include humor in daily life can protect you against emotional triggers and stressful situations. What you find funny differs from what someone else might find amusing. Therefore, you need to seek out the videos, books, television series, movies, jokes, and people that make you laugh till your stomach hurts. Keep all the things you find funny saved in a folder on your phone for easy access when needed.

Spend Time With Your Friends and Family

The power of love is taught to us by an incredibly wise 103-year-old holistic medicine doctor, Dr. Gladys McGary. "These five Ls help to structure what I'm doing, and the center of it all is love," she says.

Love is the nourishment that the other Ls require.

- Life and love are one unit. You can't have one without the other.
- Laugher with love is joy and happiness.
- Labor with love is bliss; it's why you do what you do.
- Listening with love is understanding, which enriches our lives by deepening our social bonds and allowing us to gain new perspectives.

Humans are wired for social connection, so when you spend time with those you love, you feel a sense of safety and pure joy. Research indicates that isolating yourself from your social circle and spending more time alone increases anxiety and depression. Spend time with your friends and family, and don't avoid or decline invites to social gatherings. You can cherish these precious moments forever, making you smile and feel loved. Note that you don't need to spend every minute you have available with your loved ones. Make time to fulfill your social needs and recharge your energy by taking time for yourself. The beauty is in the balance.

Attend Therapy Sessions

If you notice that you cannot regulate your emotions independently, consider seeing a therapist who can help you learn emotional regulation skills. It may take time to fully utilize all the tools available to regulate your emotions effectively. Benefiting from the tools will need your cooperation and effort. You may not feel motivated alone, but a therapist will help you every step of the way. Therapists also hold your hand on your healing journey and assist you when they can by guiding, offering support, and showing you new ways of thinking.

Here is the story of a survivor who learned to stay calm in triggering situations and reclaimed her life (Madly Calm, n.d.):

"Being an anxious person with an overactive mind, learning breathing techniques to control my nervous system has had a huge impact on my health," she stated. She has been able to retrain her thinking process and re-educate her emotions to turn the dial down. Regulating her feelings has been vital to her overall well-being.

Breathing practices provided dramatic and subtle benefits to many areas of her life: improved relationships, patience, renewed energy, and the ability to reset, control, and balance my emotions.

She stated, "My life has always been filled with doing for others, but in the past eighteen months, I have flipped the switch and started to look after myself."

INTERACTIVE ELEMENT

The Interactive Elements Workbook for Chapter 6 offers a Self-Assessment Quiz to evaluate your current emotional regulation skills. Use it for your own self-reflection to decide which areas need your attention.

SEGUE

With improved emotional control, you will move on to explore how to process your past in Chapter 7.

7

PROCESSING THE PAST

> *I have great respect for the past. If you don't know where you've come from, you don't know where you're going. I have respect for the past, but I'm a person of the moment. I'm here, and I do my best to be completely centered at the place I'm at, and then I go forward to the next place.*

— MAYA ANGELOU

Maya Angelou's quote teaches us that the past provides lessons to propel us in life. Know and understand your past to move forward. The quote lets you know that your past is your past, your presence is needed in the present, and you can move forward when you are grounded in the moment. Don't be controlled by your past; control how your past will impact the present and future. By confronting your past traumas, you take charge of what happened and its effect on you. If you ignore past trauma, it will unconsciously control your whole life. You will not be in control; your past will take the wheel and steer the ship.

Next is the story of Kiersten Johnson, who suffered from CPTSD (Johnson, n.d.):

After several years of erratic behavior, including late-night drinking, emotionally unavailable relationships, and angry outbursts, Kiersten Johnson finally sought help. "No more late nights as I am unable to take all the emotional build-up and deciding instead to go out drinking until I blacked out. No more taking my hairpins and scraping them across my knees to find relief. No more chasing after people who only used me as a scapegoat. No more screaming at innocent people just because they wanted to help. No. More."

Kiersten discussed these realizations with her grandmother after a long bout with self-harm, confessing her struggles and expressing her desire for a change. "I didn't want to live the way I was living anymore. I wanted out. I had hit rock bottom, although I didn't want to end my life; I wanted this nightmare to stop." Her parents seemed indifferent to her health, and her partner's main concern was that she wasn't confiding in him about her problems.

After careful deliberation, Kiersten's grandmother accompanied her to a mental health facility, where she spoke with a professional. Immediately, Kiersten answered affirmatively to the question, "Have you thought about hurting yourself or anyone else in the past forty-eight hours?" Fortunately, she was selected for outpatient care, requiring twice-weekly sessions with a psychologist. The set of rules included mandatory talk therapy and staying under her grandmother's care. The mental health facility also conducted random check-ins.

Talk therapy initially felt grueling for Kiersten. "I hated it at first. My therapist was a wonderful woman who did everything she could think of to get me to open up." The process took time and tremendous effort. Some days, Kiersten was willing to talk about her past, while screams and accusations marked others. Despite the challenges, her therapist saw progress as long as she wasn't sitting in silence like in the initial sessions. Even today, Kiersten continues to see a therapist to maintain her progress.

Looking through the window of Kiersten's life today reveals a transformed individual. "I take medication for my depression and anxiety. I do somatic breathing techniques with my yoga, which is highly recommended for anyone with PTSD." She left her soul-crushing job to become a full-time writer, taking things slowly and carefully. In other words, she now cares for herself like she wished someone had done when she was young.

In this chapter, you will delve into confronting and processing your past traumas, focusing on healing and letting go.

BENEFITS OF CONFRONTING YOUR PAST TRAUMAS

Living with unresolved trauma impacts every area of your life. You struggle to maintain relationships. You are disappointed, betrayed, or become anxiously attached. Romantic relationships and friendships never seem to last long in your life. Work life becomes stressful as you lack boundaries and allow others to walk all over you. Or, perhaps you're stuck in an unfulfilling job or relationship, but you don't make a move to change your situation. Maybe you use work as your coping strategy, where you drown yourself in your job to escape the pain of your emotional wounds.

Do you hold back in your relationships to avoid feeling vulnerable? The world doesn't feel like a pleasant place to live when you are dealing with unresolved trauma. Your past traumas can hold you back from living the life you truly deserve.

You often notice being at war with yourself and engaging in habits you don't enjoy as an escape, but you are unsure why. The answer to your behavior is unprocessed trauma that occurred sometime in your life that might have been suppressed or forgotten.

Sometimes, events seem irrelevant and not as impactful until you reach a certain age or phase. For example, a girl was sexually harassed at the age of 19 by her boss—a man who could be the same age as her father. She decided to further her studies and later on became a therapist. She never reported the incident or told anybody, believing she was okay. But, when she experienced panic attacks before seeing clients, she realized something was not right. She and her therapist analyzed the situation together. They discovered that before seeing a male client who is older than 50 years old, she would go into panic mode. It took her back to the 19-year-old version of herself who couldn't protect or stand up to her boss. Her body remembered, but her mind didn't recall the sexual harassment case.

Your brain draws on past experiences and knowledge to guide you. Think of your brain as a master of connections and patterns, a repository of collective wisdom. Your past experiences and lessons learned shape your gut instinct, offering you insights and feelings, whether good or bad. Your gut feeling is wisdom based on what you've experienced and learned.

So, be careful. Reacting from your gut can separate you from your heart. Because when you respond from your gut, you could be reacting from fear. It's a memory response rooted in trauma. Your mind doesn't always recall the memories of the past. Still, the trauma is stored in your nervous system, and your body keeps a record of everything that has ever happened to you. Confronting your traumas allows you to grow and let go of the past. It helps you to act from the conscious mind and not to be controlled by your unconscious mind.

Here is a list of the benefits of facing your past traumas:

- You start to see that you are strong enough to overcome obstacles in life.
- You can build authentic and stronger interpersonal connections.
- You increase your ability to be resilient.
- You build a stronger bond with yourself.
- You begin to understand why you act the way you do.

Face the Pain

Confronting your past seems anxiety-provoking. You must deliberately put yourself in the challenging situation of returning to old hurtful memories and unpleasant emotions. You have to go back to the past to move on from your trauma. Facing your pain doesn't seem ideal at the moment, but your future self will thank you for doing so.

You have heard the saying, "There's no rainbow without rain," and the same goes for healing from your past. First, you will experience pain by going through the storm, facing the obstacles and tribulations, learning the lessons the past wants to teach you, and eventually working on letting your past go. When you heal your emotional wounds and let go of your past, the storm stops, and you can see the rainbow.

Lessons From the Past

The evidence suggests that life situations cannot be ignored and that we cannot move on from hurt until we have learned every lesson it was meant to teach us. Every problem can be understood by viewing every experience as an educational opportunity. To do so, we must be open to receiving the lessons.

We should become curious about our past and present experiences and look for their meaning. It is essential to look at things at face value, dig deeper, and find the hidden lessons. You may be surprised by the valuable insights you can gain from past traumas. You can learn more from your past experiences than from a motivational speaker or guru. One of the best ways to heal from your past is to take the lessons you have learned and use them to enhance your growth.

Let Go of the Past

Letting go of your past and healing from your trauma is bittersweet for some trauma survivors. As mentioned before, after a traumatic experience, you become a new person as a result of the impact the traumatic event had on you. This identity you formed to adapt to the world post-trauma is comfortable.

Healing allows you to create a new and improved identity. However, for trauma survivors, the unknown is scary, so they will choose to stick to an identity centered around trauma. That can be all they know; the familiar makes them feel comfortable.

To completely detach from trauma and move on, this list of strategies highlights opportunities to help you let go of the past:

- Create a positive affirmation for every negative thought each time emotional wounds trigger you.
- Distance yourself physically and psychologically from the trauma.
- Name five things you are grateful for when you experience flashbacks or triggered thoughts.
- Engage in mindfulness activities daily.
- Practice compassion for yourself and others.
- Allow yourself to feel all emotions, positive and negative.
- Accept that the person involved in your traumatizing experience may never apologize.
- Prioritize regular self-care.
- Spend time with people who add meaning to your life.
- Allow yourself to vent when life feels too overwhelming.

Practice Forgiveness

Forgiveness is a powerful act that holds immense personal benefits and frees the forgiver and the forgiven. When we choose to forgive, we unburden ourselves from anger, resentment, and bitterness. While forgiveness may not always be easy, especially in the face of deep hurt or wrongdoing, it allows us to shed the past and stride forward with a heart brimming with love and compassion.

Forgiveness is not a passive act of condoning or forgetting the hurt caused by others. It is a conscious decision to release the negative emotions that shackle us, preventing us from experiencing true peace and joy. It is a choice to extend grace and mercy, freeing us from the grievances that weigh on our hearts.

Let us cultivate a spirit of forgiveness and experience freedom and healing. Consider how different life might look and feel if you could:

- Talk about your past trauma without triggering or distressing you.
- Feel peace and grace toward the person or event that traumatized you.

"Forgive yourself and the ones who harmed you" is easier said than done. Sometimes, you want to forgive someone but just can't do it. Other times, you may refuse to forgive another person, as this gives you a sense of control. What they did was hurtful and caused you years of living with trauma.

What are some practical steps one can take to forgive someone who has caused trauma?

The key is to recognize that forgiveness is more about you and less about the other person. Forgiveness lets you release anger, resentment, and lingering feelings about a situation, positively impacting your well-being and relationships with others.

Here are seven benefits of forgiving others:

- You feel less anxious.
- You feel an increased sense of empowerment.
- You become more hopeful about life.
- You treat others with kindness.
- Your heart health will improve.
- Your quality of sleep improves.
- Your immune system becomes stronger.

Remember to forgive yourself when practicing forgiveness, as you are the most important person to forgive. Forgive yourself for the decisions you have made and your emotional responses while you were in survival mode. Forgive yourself for all the times you told yourself, "I should have known." Forgive yourself for releasing the negative emotions you direct at yourself and letting go of beliefs that sabotage your well-being.

Forgive yourself for allowing other people to affect your sense of self-worth. I recall a time when I let tarnished relationships impact my life. I felt an innate need for approval from those who shut me out. I asked myself, "Why do I allow others to influence my behavior?" I recognized this as a trait in my personality. Acting on my heart's desires, I reached out to repair relationships but received no response. I realized that I needed validation to know my self-worth.

The reality is that those relationships were toxic and served only to cause me more pain. After years of trying to make amends, I let go. My life is peaceful as I am surrounded by people who share my joys and pain.

Perhaps you've felt let down by someone you care about or even allowed these experiences to shape how you see yourself. It's natural to feel disappointed or let down when someone we care about doesn't show up for us how we need them to.

But it's important to remember that their behavior is a reflection of them, not of you. You cannot control others; you can only control your reaction to them. Relationships are two-way, so you can control your next steps if one is not giving back to you or has disappointed you.

You are worthy of love and respect, no matter what others do or don't do. Accepting when someone you care about does not reciprocate or acknowledge you is challenging. They refuse to share their life with you. Can you disconnect and let it go?

The answer is you can.

The path forward is forgiving yourself for allowing others to affect your self-worth. It is an essential step on the path to self-love. Forgiving yourself will enable you to release the pain of the past and focus on creating healthy, loving relationships in the present. It opens up the possibility of healing and happiness.

SELF-HELP THERAPEUTIC TECHNIQUES

In this section, you will gain knowledge and tips for processing the past through healing the inner child and engaging in shadow work. Both these strategies are effective therapeutic techniques for healing from the past.

Heal the Inner Child

Healing is so hard because it is a constant battle between your inner child, who is scared and just wants safety, and your current self, who is tired and just wants peace. No matter your age, you will always have an inner child. The inner child is a sub-personality that lives in your subconscious and holds emotions, memories, and beliefs from the past. The inner child can be of various ages as it represents multiple events in your childhood. The wounded inner child is believed to be the age at which it became traumatized or wounded. If you were bullied at school at the age of six, your wounded inner child will be six years old.

Inner child work is a therapeutic technique that aids in identifying and healing trauma that occurred during childhood. It will help you understand your behavior, emotional triggers, and needs as an adult. Inner child work allows you to go back to the past, dig for information, and reparent your inner child by giving it the love and care it never received. As an adult, you will try your best to meet the needs of the wounded inner child.

Here are a few signs that your inner child may be wounded and crying out for help:

- You become frustrated or irritated easily.
- You throw tantrums when your needs go unmet.
- When you are triggered, you say things you don't mean.
- You frequently feel misunderstood and unheard.
- You struggle to articulate your emotions or convey the complexities of your inner world.
- You battle with low self-esteem.
- You deal with cruel and harmful self-talk.
- Others often say you are immature.
- You often engage in self-sabotaging acts.
- You have a fear of being abandoned.
- You need more boundaries, or they could be more assertive.
- You have unhealthy coping skills.

Healing the wounded inner child is a different approach to healing from the past. You heal from childhood trauma that impacts you today by healing the inner child. The wounded inner child can disrupt your adult world and lead you to destructive and self-sabotaging behaviors. The wounded inner child has a strong hold on you as an adult and gets away with many adverse decisions. Your wounded inner child is the constant voice that keeps nagging you to do bad things.

Let's say the wounded inner child has been bullied and laughed at during oral presentations at school. As an adult, the wounded inner child tries to bombard you with old beliefs when giving presentations at work. When you give the presentation, the wounded inner child experiences the same feelings of being tormented when you were younger.

Healing the wounded inner child can help you reconnect with your passions, dreams, and hobbies. It can give you the confidence to unleash your talents and tap into parts of yourself that you may have been afraid to share. As a result, you start feeling empowered and in control of your life. Healing the wounded inner child can also help you make healthier decisions and improve your emotional regulation skills. To heal the wounded inner child, you must update her belief system, soothe her overwhelming emotions, and meet her needs just as a loving mother would tend to her distressed child. While you may not have control over your past, you can break free from its hold on you.

Start healing the wounded inner child with these tips:

- **Pay attention to the inner child:** Start listening to your inner child. What is the inner child telling you when you feel emotional? What does the inner child need? Make the wounded inner child feel heard and understood.
- **Practice meditation:** Meditation helps create a safe space for your inner child to experience all emotions. You may have been rejected, shamed, or scolded in childhood for showing anger or crying. Your wounded inner child believes, "I am not allowed to feel angry or sad." With meditation, you teach your wounded inner child that feeling negative emotions is okay and safe.
- **Be your parent:** Working to heal your inner child helps you realize that your parents were not perfect and only did the best they knew how. Now it's your turn to take full responsibility for your wounded inner child and meet her

needs, show her love, and make decisions in her best interest. Reparenting your inner child is about unlearning the destructive habits, behaviors, and beliefs you picked up during childhood. You can practice self-care and compassion as the new caregiver of your wounded inner child. Furthermore, next time you feel upset, try to meet your needs as you wish your parents would have done during childhood.

- **Take a trip down memory lane:** Have you ever wondered why your inner child may be wounded? Reflect on your childhood memories to gain insights into the causes. Doing so lets you connect with your inner child and allows her to heal from these painful memories. Your inner child's perception of past events may be flawed. As an adult, you can develop a more accurate and realistic perspective.

- **Talk with your friends and family:** Your inner child may hold onto beliefs about family and friends from childhood. By addressing these beliefs as an adult, you can shift your perspective. Individuals you once disliked or harbored resentment towards may now be individuals you appreciate. This process can give you a deeper comprehension of their actions and choices during your formative years, facilitating the release of past traumas. Opening up to family and friends can aid in achieving closure.

- **Allow yourself to have fun:** Connect with your inner child by listening to and asking about her favorite hobby or game. Use the answer to start playing and having fun again. Part of healing is having fun and making yourself happy.

Shadow Work

> Until you make the unconscious conscious, it will direct your life, and you will call it fate.

— CARL JUNG

Everyone has a side of themselves hidden from the world. This part is the shadow self, which can be described as the darker, less acceptable aspects of one's personality. According to Carl Jung, the shadow self comprises the inferior, immoral, and emotional parts of one's being.

You may feel insecure about these traits and may have even been teased or criticized for them. For example, if you were a talkative child, someone may have told you that you talked too much, giving them a headache. Comments like these can cause you to hide certain parts of your personality from others.

The shadow self is the part of you that gets repressed and forgotten. Repressing your shadow leads to dangerous consequences. By hiding the shadow self, you are unable to live authentically. Your shadow self surfaces when you are emotionally triggered. It comes to light when you believe you are acting out of character or out of pocket. When the emotions subside, you realize that your shadow slipped and manifested on the surface for others to see. You may regret it and later be embarrassed.

By doing shadow work, you discover all the parts you have hidden, which could be a traumatic event or undesirable parts of your personality. The main goal of shadow work is to become self-aware and to practice self-acceptance. Shadow work aids in processing trauma to embrace and show love to the parts of you that have been suppressed and shamed.

Practical Shadow Work Exercises

The following three exercises focus on identifying your shadow self and learning to accept and embrace all the unlikeable parts of yourself.

Think About Someone You Dislike

Exploring the individuals who trigger strong negative emotions within you can illuminate your shadow side. Delve deeper into understanding these individuals by reflecting on the following inquiries:

1. Which specific qualities about this person evoke my dislike?
2. What additional personality traits are shared between this individual and me?
3. What challenges do I encounter when in their presence?
4. Which aspects of my character become prominent when interacting with them?

Exploring these questions can reveal aspects of your shadow self. It is a common belief that the traits we dislike in others may also reside within our own shadows. These traits are not necessarily harmful, as the other person may cherish these parts of themselves. You may feel triggered because you have rejected these traits and hidden them away in your shadow out of shame.

Analyze Your Family

Make a family tree and be honest about each family member. Below each individual, write down their personality traits. Avoid sugar-coating anybody's life or personality.

Identify specific behaviors or actions that you find displeasing or elicit strong emotional reactions. After pinpointing these aspects, reflect on whether or not you possess similar or identical traits.

Face Your Shadow

The previous two exercises can help you identify various parts of your shadow self. In this third exercise, you will face your shadow self during meditation. While meditating, think of one personality trait or insecurity you have repressed for years. Say a positive affirmation that aims to release the shadow self.

Here are examples of positive affirmations:

- I allow the darkest parts of me to be released.
- I let go of my shame, fears, and insecurities.
- I am worthy of love and respect just as I am.
- I trust in my abilities and believe in my potential to succeed.
- I embrace my imperfections as they make me unique and special.
- I release all negative self-talk and replace it with positivity and self-love.
- I am confident, capable, and deserving of all life's goodness.
- This quality has probably served me at some point, but I no longer need this protection. I release this trait or insecurity from my shadows.

Remember, practicing these daily affirmations can help rewire your mindset and empower you to overcome insecurities. I'm cheering you on!

GUIDANCE TO FIND HELP FROM MENTAL HEALTH PRACTITIONERS

While the book may offer insights and perspectives on well-being, it is not a substitute for professional therapeutic advice or treatment. Therapists trained in trauma can provide insight and depth in a safe and supportive way. They won't leave you wallowing in deep feelings.

Finding the right mental health practitioner is essential to your healing journey. If you are new to the mental health world, don't fret! This section will help you find the right practitioner for you.

Before finding the best mental health practitioner, ask yourself these questions:

- What are my goals?
- What is my budget?
- Who can I ask for recommendations?
- Which local resources are available in my area?

Knowing what you want to achieve is the best way to seek help from a mental health practitioner. You and the therapist become a team and work together to achieve your goals. Therefore, it's crucial to approach therapy with clear objectives and a distinct understanding of the areas in which you need help.

Create a budget for your mental health, or contact your insurance company to determine your options. If you cannot afford the fees, ask friends, family, or your doctor to recommend affordable mental health practitioners or places that offer free therapy. Your place of worship, workplace, or school may provide mental health services free of charge.

Therapy or support groups can speed up your healing process in many ways. Therapy can offer you support and guidance, equip you with healthy coping mechanisms, and educate you about trauma. Therapy and support groups give you a safe space to share your story without judgment. It's a space where you can be your authentic self, and you will find others with similar experiences and problems. This support makes you feel less alone and understood. Your well-being will benefit from regular therapy or support group sessions.

How do you know the best mental health practitioner for you? Finding the best option is personal, as you won't feel comfortable with just any therapist or support group. To avoid awkwardness and disappointment, ensure you know the answers to the following questions about the practitioner you choose:

- Are they licensed or registered to practice in your state?
- How many years have they been practicing?
- How much experience do they have dealing with a client's trauma?
- What is their specialty?
- What treatment or techniques do they find compelling to treat trauma?
- Do you feel seen, heard, and respected when talking to them?
- Do they demonstrate excellent listening skills?
- Are they able to show empathy and emotional support?
- Do you feel they invalidate your feelings?

- Are they punctual?
- Are they fully present during your session?

These questions will help you identify red flags. You can ask around and read their online reviews. If you like the self-help techniques offered in this book, you may enjoy a therapist who also utilizes them. Choose a mental health practitioner wisely, as it's essential for your healing journey and future.

INTERACTIVE ELEMENT

The Free Interactive Elements Workbook includes a Journaling Exercise for Chapter 7 to begin processing your traumatic experiences. Use the prompts provided to help you start your journaling exercise. When you are ready, move on to Chapter 8.

Segue

With a better understanding of your past, you will explore resilience and persistence in Chapter 8.

8

STAND IN YOUR POWER

> *Mastering others is strength. Mastering yourself is true power.*
>
> — LAO TZU

It is essential not to be impacted by others' words and actions and to overcome the negative voice in your head. Some days, it may be easy to shake another person's words, but fighting your thoughts isn't always straightforward. You stand in your true power when you win the battle against your emotional wounds, insecurities, and negative thoughts.

Here is the story of a survivor who reclaimed her power after trauma (Rainn, n.d.):

After enduring 13 years of struggle with emotional, financial, spiritual, and sexual abuse, Courageous was determined to shield her daughters from their abuser, her then-husband. She thought, "Maybe I'm crazy, maybe we keep misunderstanding each other, or maybe we are right at the brink of a breakthrough." As time passed, she expressed, "My kids and I were determined to keep making space to be with each other even though he tried to put so much conflict between us."

When her abuser finally exited her life and with potential family court involvement and the possibility of her children being forced into visitation on the horizon, Courageous desired to educate her children about the emotional abuse they had all endured. She wanted her daughters to possess the language to comprehend the manipulation and control they had experienced.

By educating her daughters on the technical definitions of different types of abuse and prompting them to reflect on their personal experiences, she empowered them to link these definitions with specific behaviors. This teaching enabled them to understand the harm they were being shielded from and recognize that the harm's source was the individual perpetrating it. Recalling her daughters asking, "Well, mom, what did he do to you? What's that called?" She answered their questions even though her daughters were just 10 and 12 at the time, "It was important that they felt fully informed from now on with nothing hidden."

Courageous channeled her experience into advocacy, educating, and empowering her Black community about domestic violence. Recognizing a lack of awareness where the misconception persisted that abuse only involved physical violence, she founded Courageous Fire, LLC, to create safe spaces and provide education to Black women. While her initial focus was on domestic violence survivors, Courageous shifted her work to include Black women in crisis, as abuse can encompass many forms of violence and trauma.

After 13 years, Courageous emerged from a self-sabotaging thinking pattern that made her believe she was at fault. Reflecting on her journey, "Trauma causes your internal world to turn against you, shut off your needs, resulting in self-sabotage." To empower oneself, she emphasizes the need to overlook traumatic thoughts and beliefs by starting to acknowledge strengths. Courageous invites others to embrace their inner strength and self-empowerment as they continue their healing journey.

In this chapter, you will learn to embrace your inner strength and self-empowerment as you continue your healing journey.

PERSONAL EMPOWERMENT

Traumatic events can completely disrupt your world and leave you feeling stuck. Following such experiences, you might find yourself adrift, lacking motivation, feeling trapped, and grappling with diminished self-worth. It's easy to get trapped in a cycle of negativity, making it challenging to view life through a positive lens.

It may seem like you've hit rock bottom and transformed into a different version of yourself. However, it's crucial not to let rock bottom become your comfort zone. Remember, you don't have to endure the negative aftermath of trauma indefinitely.

It's common for trauma survivors to express a sense of profound transformation. Regaining a sense of empowerment and boosting your confidence is well within your grasp. Recovery from trauma is not only feasible but also a journey towards healing and growth.

To recover from trauma, you need the courage to step out of the negative rut and empower yourself. Personal empowerment is a great tool for healing from trauma. Enduring trauma and all the negative emotions that come with it leads to feeling unmotivated to do things that make you feel empowered. Healing starts with you. You can begin by taking small steps on your healing journey using self-help methods. You learn to take control of your life and reclaim your power by empowering yourself. Personal empowerment involves making positive choices that will benefit your future self.

Loving yourself is a vital tool to become an empowered individual. When you begin the journey to wellness after trauma, you will learn to love yourself enough to help you climb the mountain to find the healed version of you. Personal empowerment is essential on your healing journey as it takes you from rock bottom to a point where you want to recover, overcome your trauma, and create a life you love.

Strategies to Empower Yourself

In this section, we look at methods to deal with trauma denial, dismissiveness, toxic positivity, and aggression. These four aspects are natural responses to trauma to protect yourself from the emotional pain caused by a traumatic event.

Trauma Denial and Dismissiveness

Denial serves as a protective mechanism employed by individuals to safeguard against confronting emotional distress that they may not be prepared to address. Denial is your brain trying to adapt to your system overloaded with new, threatening, and overwhelming information. Being in denial about the traumatic event isn't always a planned decision; it is an automatic response after trauma. Denial is a short-term method to cope as it minimizes the impact of trauma on your well-being. In denial, you continue living life as usual, create a false sense of control, protect your self-esteem, and carry on in a relationship with someone who hurt you.

The more you depend on using denial as a crutch, the more suffering you will endure. Denial involves suppressing a traumatic event, indicating that the brain is reluctant to address it immediately, leading to the mind and body eventually confronting the repercussions.

Confronting your trauma face-to-face is scary and may create intense fear. Can you imagine anyone who consciously wants to engage in hurtful memories that cause an emotional wound? Therefore, trauma denial is a better option in the moment. The healed version of you is waiting on the other side of denial.

Overcome trauma denial and dismissiveness with self-care techniques, including:

• Practice yoga	• Undergo somatic healing
• Complete breathing exercises	• Read trauma recovery books
• Perform grounding activities	• Enjoy massage therapy
• Engage in regular exercise	• Participate in daily meditation

Toxic Positivity

This empowerment aspect refers to a belief that you must remain positive, even in a traumatizing or stressful situation. You force yourself into only thinking positive thoughts and being optimistic about life. Positive thinking is an excellent approach to life and benefits your well-being. Still, when it becomes toxic, you start to reject the negative parts of life and paint them as positive. Toxic positivity distorts your reality. It makes you ignore all negative emotions to experience happiness. You may engage in toxic positivity to deal with difficult life situations. However, it is not a healthy and practical coping skill.

Toxic positivity minimizes and denies any experience that doesn't fall under the optimistic and happy category. Many people live by the quote, "Good vibes only." Many well-meaning people encourage you to engage in toxic positivity by saying,

- "Stay positive, my friend!"
- "But look on the bright side."
- "Everything happens for a reason."
- "Just think happy thoughts."
- "Focus on the good."
- "Happiness is a choice."

The phrases come from a good place but can make you feel rejected and misunderstood, increase feelings of hurt, and, in some cases, cause you to shut down. The people who respond in these ways are likely afraid of experiencing their own negative emotions and so rely on toxic positivity to distract themselves from their own fear, sadness, grief, etc.

Toxic positivity blocks you from growth, development, and healing. Life can never be *good vibes only* because life is about living and learning. Life is never all sunshine and roses. You will endure unpleasant experiences because they are part of the human experience. Instead of engaging in toxic positivity, deal with your emotions and experiences openly so that you learn to accept and effectively work through them. You may even realize that life's unpleasant feelings are simple guidance to alert you that something is amiss. Refer back to Chapter 5 to review the hidden messages of emotions.

To let go of engaging in toxic positivity, try these methods:

- Develop a mindset that makes it okay not to be okay.
- Self-soothe unpleasant emotions.

- Become more realistic when experiencing negative experiences.
- Permit yourself to feel negative emotions.
- Teach yourself that negative and positive emotions can occur simultaneously.
- Be curious about the meaning of your experiences.
- Unfollow social media accounts that preach toxic positivity.
- Give your feelings a voice.
- Validate your emotions.

Aggression

It's normal to have an intense emotional and physical response to trauma. It's human instinct to react strongly when distressed. Aggression is a typical result of trauma.

It can be challenging to control your response while in survivor mode; you may become aggressive as your nervous system fights against the traumatic experience that activated your flight-or-fight-or-freeze response. Your automatic reaction and intense emotions will subside within seconds to minutes as the body starts calming down.

During trauma recovery, your body may be in a prolonged state of flight-or-fight-or-freeze mode, which causes you to act aggressively toward others. You become sensitive and ready to pounce when they say something you don't like. When you get over the trauma and heal your nervous system, you leave survival mode, feeling more relaxed.

To manage your aggression during survival mode, try the following:

- Choose your battles wisely; learn when to engage and which to ignore.
- Avoid spending your energy on irrelevant matters.
- Communicate your emotions constructively and assertively.
- Do activities that help you restore emotional energy.
- Talk yourself through moments where your nervous system is activated.
- Avoid being hyper-focused on the negatives.
- Use physical activity (burpees, lunches, or jogging) to let those emotions flow through you and out.
- Do not attempt to suppress your feelings, only your behaviors. Do not speak to or touch another person while angry.
- Take a time-out for yourself. If you are a parent, this could mean spending extra time in the bathroom, so long as your kids are in a safe space.
- Try narrative therapy by journalling or speaking aloud without judgment about the sensations and emotions that arise. Once this feels complete, you can reframe and write this story for yourself.

WHO DO YOU TELL?

Your trauma story isn't something you share with just anybody. When you begin to heal, you may want to talk about your trauma to someone. Or you may be closed off from letting someone into your inner world. The thought of being vulnerable around others can bring fear and anxiety if you fear that they will shame, dismiss, deny, reject, or give you a guilt trip.

Here is the story of a survivor who opened up about sexual assault for the first time:

When she first opened up to a high school boyfriend about her childhood sexual assault, she was met with disgust. "Eventually, he even held the assault over my head as a form of blackmail during an argument, threatening to tell the entire school — as if I should feel ashamed," she recalls.

This experience made her vow never to share her trauma again. However, deep down, she knew she had simply confided in the wrong person. "I knew those closest to me would love, respect, and support me if I explained what had happened and how it impacted me presently," she reflects. Eventually, she found the courage to speak up again. "It was through doing so that I shed my shame, built a supportive community, and began to heal."

They might blame you and make you feel like you're at fault for the trauma you have experienced instead of supporting you. This fear of everyone's reaction can drive trauma survivors to take their experience to their grave, never experiencing the love and support they long for. Trauma is no longer a taboo subject. Lots of support and love are waiting for you.

Empowerment in trauma recovery is accepting what happened, owning your story, and retelling it to others when you are ready. Trauma should not be kept a secret as it decreases the chances of healing, which could lead to suppressed emotions manifesting during unwanted moments. To heal does not mean you need to have a family meeting and tell them about your traumatic experience.

When you tell your story, choose a loyal and trusted person you know can emotionally support you. The person can be a trusted family member, a friend, or a mental health practitioner. The person you tell can offer a new perspective, guide you to different avenues for help, and provide support. You don't have to go through difficult experiences on your own. Sharing your story is a liberating experience that lightens the weight of bearing the traumatic event alone, enabling you to progress forward.

Keep in mind that sharing your story is optional. The choice is entirely yours. Remember, you are the hero in your life story. How do you want to write it?

SELF-ADVOCACY

Empowerment includes advocating for yourself. Self-advocacy is letting your voice be heard by speaking up for yourself. In trauma recovery, self-advocacy is standing in your power and letting others know how to support you. Advocating for yourself means identifying and sharing your needs with others using assertive and clear communication.

In your healing journey, it's essential to communicate how others can best support, motivate, and guide you. Equally crucial is outlining behaviors that may inadvertently contribute to your trauma and distress. While not everyone may naturally exhibit the empathy and kindness you seek, educating those around you on how to interact with sensitivity is essential. While expecting everyone to tiptoe around you is unrealistic, fostering an environment of consideration and emotional support can make a significant difference in your healing process.

You must communicate your expectations so others know how to fulfill your needs. You cannot expect others to understand what you are going through if you do not inform them. Here is a story about Belinda.

Belinda gets angry and feels her feelings are not considered at family gatherings. She believes her family didn't support her through the difficult breakup with her boyfriend. At family gatherings, her aunts ask Belinda, "When are you and Brad getting married?" This question makes her want to scream. She never told anybody about the break-up, only her older sister. Belinda also never tells her aunts that she doesn't like the question; instead, she lies and cracks jokes.

Learning to advocate for yourself avoids many unwanted, awkward, and heated situations in the future. Communicating your needs lets others know what to say. Avoid drama by speaking up to protect your peace.

Develop your self-advocacy skills with the following tips:

- **Know your worth:** Trauma clouds your mind and makes you believe you lack respect, kindness, or support. Flip the switch and start to see your worth. You decide your worthiness, not your past experiences or people. Believe you are worthy of being treated with kindness, respect, empathy, and love.
- **Identify your weaknesses:** Your vulnerabilities provide insight for growth and will indicate what you can and cannot tolerate. You may be tempted to create a boundary around the attributes you see as your weaknesses. However, being aware of your weaknesses can help you prepare for or avoid certain situations.
- **Increase your confidence:** Someone who never speaks up for herself and just goes with the flow likely has low confidence. You may be allowing others to walk all over you and hurt you. Working to elevate your self-confidence will increase your ability to advocate for yourself.

- **Challenge your inner voice:** Trauma can turn your inner voice against you, filling your mind with false beliefs about yourself. This negative self-talk can breed feelings of insecurity and diminish your self-esteem. It's crucial to confront this inner voice head-on or, at times, simply tune it out. Challenging or disregarding these detrimental thoughts can boost your self-esteem and empower you to advocate for your well-being.
- **Communicate your needs early:** Telling or showing others how you want to be treated should be done early in a relationship as it eliminates future disappointments and misunderstandings. Communication allows relationships to flourish, enabling you to feel loved and supported. When others respect your needs, you feel emotionally safe to speak up.

Protect Your Boundaries

As a trauma survivor, boundaries are essential to protect your internal world from your external world. Boundaries are the limits you set around your physical body, belongings, time, energy, and mental health. Your boundaries are the rules you set for others who want to step into your life. Boundaries make you feel empowered, prevent others from taking advantage of you, and prevent you from being mentally drained and manipulated by others. Without boundaries, your internal world will crumble. Others can hurt you whether they intend to or not. Not having boundaries tends to make you lose yourself in things you are passionate about, such as your relationships or career. Healthy and consistent boundaries, on the other hand, increase your self-esteem and aid in lowering stress levels.

You can start by identifying the areas of your life to set boundaries. You can begin with these ideas:

- Emotional energy
- Time
- Personal space
- Sexuality
- Morals and ethics
- Values and beliefs
- Material possessions and finances
- Social media

Establishing boundaries empowers you to say "no" without guilt. Many trauma survivors grapple with this issue. Have you ever encountered someone who consistently agrees, even at their own expense? This immediate acquiescence could indicate a lack of solid boundaries. It's crucial to understand that expressing disagreement or refusal isn't impolite and doesn't warrant an apology. Societal conditioning often makes us feel remorse for uttering a simple "no." However, it's a form of self-love and a testament to respecting your boundaries. Always align your responses with your instinctual feelings. If your intuition encourages a "yes," embrace it. Conversely, if it signals a "no," respect your feelings and confidently express your refusal.

Here are some strategies to help you say no to others:

- **Replace the word "no"** with "I'll get back to you with an answer later."
- **Practice saying "no"** with role play in the mirror.
- **Pause** before answering a question.

- **Be clear and concise** without explanation when saying "no."
- **Avoid offering an alternative**; just say "no."
- **Ensure that your body language** aligns with the message you are conveying.

Consider these tips to ensure that your body language aligns with your words:

- **Maintain Eye Contact** to show your engagement and interest in the conversation. It also helps to build trust and connection.
- **Use an Open Posture** by facing the individual to demonstrate your receptiveness to their input.
- **Use Gestures Appropriately** with hand gestures to help emphasize your points and enthusiasm.
- **Control Your Facial Expressions** by practicing to control your facial expressions to align your true feelings with your words.
- **Monitor Your Voice** to keep your tone consistent with your message, as it says much about your feelings.
- **Respect Personal Space** by honoring the other person's space to ensure comfort and mutual understanding.

Remember, body language is a skill that can be improved with practice. So, keep these tips in mind and practice them regularly.

Dealing with Disregard of Boundaries

What occurs when individuals disregard your boundaries and persistently reject your refusal?

Occasionally, you may find people challenging your limits. However, it's your responsibility to maintain these boundaries, not theirs. Consider it like safeguarding your personal property and its perimeters. Defending your territory against those who wish to intrude without consent is crucial. Establishing boundaries also necessitates setting consequences for those who disrespect them. To ensure your boundaries are honored, you must take proactive measures to protect them.

To protect against violating your boundaries, identify and under-stand your boundaries. Then, you need to communicate those boundaries to others. Ensure you are clear, direct, and confident at this moment.

Your boundaries should not be too rigid and can differ from person to person. So, what do you do when someone crosses your boundaries?

Your boundaries need to be realistic so you can stand by them. Your friend, who is always late for everything, has planned a lunch date with you. You told her you would leave after waiting 10 minutes, but you still sit at the restaurant 20 minutes later. By doing this, you are not protecting your boundaries. Protect your boundaries by following through precisely as you said you would.

INTERACTIVE ELEMENT

The Chapter 8 Interactive Element includes a Self-Assessment Activity to identify your unique sources of personal power and a Build Your Strengths Exercise to identify and cultivate your strengths. You'll find it in the Free Interactive Elements Workbook.

SEGUE

Now that you have learned about self-empowerment, you can move on with creating your vision in Chapter 9.

9

A VISION OF SOMETHING BETTER

When you combine powerful visualizations with deliberate actions, you can have whatever you seek.

— WHITNEY GORDON-MEAD

While holding onto your dreams is essential, they can only materialize through action. Constructing a purposeful and fulfilling life is necessary for recovering from trauma and finding happiness.

Next is Kim's life story. She was inspired to find a vision of a better future (Rainn, n.d.):

In 1998, at the vulnerable age of 12, Kim's life took a dark turn when she became the target of a predatory gymnastics coach with a seemingly impeccable reputation. This sinister episode unfolded against the backdrop of her family grappling with her father's bipolar disorder diagnosis, creating a perfect storm of stress and turmoil that the perpetrator shamelessly exploited.

The abuse reached a horrifying crescendo during a summer gymnastics camp in a team hotel room. It wasn't until the fall of that year that the coach was finally outed for sexually assaulting three female coaching staff members, all former gymnastics students manipulated by him during their youth.

Kim's revelation didn't emerge until the following summer when she began pouring her pain into letters addressed to one of the victimized staff members. Fate intervened when her mother discovered these heart-wrenching confessions before they could be sent. Instead of resorting to legal action, Kim's family chose the path of therapy, recognizing the urgent need to address not only the abuse but also the family's internal struggles.

The therapist, regrettably, did not immediately report the abuse to the police, allowing nearly a year to pass before an investigation was launched. Despite Kim's brave disclosure, law enforcement deemed the evidence insufficient to apprehend the perpetrator. Kim grappled with the belief that her voice went unheard, her pain unnoticed, and her trauma trivialized.

A decade later, Kim uncovered a disturbing truth—her abuser had not only continued coaching but had even opened his own gym. Shockingly, he had been arrested again for sexually assaulting a child. Armed with this information, Kim reached out to the authorities, only to be informed that the statute of limitations had expired. Despite the coach's eventual conviction, he received a two-year sentence due to a plea deal shielding him as a first-time offender.

At least 11 victims shared their nightmarish experience. Learning that she was not alone offered Kim solace. Instead of succumbing to despair, she found strength in pursuing justice. Becoming a social worker in Child Protective Services in the very town where her abuse occurred, Kim stumbled upon files that validated her claims. USA Gymnastics, however, failed to acknowledge her plea until she joined a national lawsuit in 2018.

Through the legal battle, Kim connected with fellow survivors and legislators, sparking her involvement in creating legislation to protect children from sexual predators. After persistent efforts, a bill was passed, removing the criminal statute of limitations and extending the civil timeframe.

Kim's legislative endeavors empowered her and contributed to her healing process. "Being able to come forward and help save someone else is healing for me," she affirmed. Kim continues her advocacy work by championing laws protecting children from abuse. She also remains engaged in gymnastics as a coach at a local gym.

Despite the scars inflicted by her past, Kim finds purpose in ensuring that the sport, which once hurt her, becomes a haven for others. In this place, resilience triumphs over adversity. "Gymnastics hurt me, but it also saved me. After the abuse ended, the gym was my safe space, and I want to keep that going for others."

This chapter encourages you to create a vision for your future full of hope, purpose, and renewed optimism.

BUILD A MEANINGFUL LIFE

Creating a meaningful life is vital when the mind asks, "*Why was I born? What am I doing on Earth? What's the point of being alive?*"

Have you ever found yourself pondering these questions while navigating the aftermath of trauma?

The essence of life is discovered through having a clear sense of purpose in this vast world. A life devoid of meaning can lead to feelings of disorientation, heightened vulnerability, and distressing triggers. To enhance your health and well-being, embrace purpose, set meaningful goals, and uphold core values can profoundly.

What it means to live a meaningful life differs from person to person and depends on your life phase. A meaningful life serves four functions:

1. **Purpose** provides determination to give you a reason to exist, eliminating the negative questions that make you feel you have no reason to live.
2. **Congruency** aligns your behavior and actions with your meaning in life. You will cultivate standards and life values that will keep you on your righteous path.
3. **Empowerment** allows you to control uncomfortable events in your life.
4. **Self-worth** increases your feelings of worthiness and helps you find a new version of yourself.

To envision a future filled with personal growth, fulfillment, and meaningful experiences, use the following strategies:

- **Find your purpose in life** by exploring your passion and what fulfills you. Finding your purpose could be a dream you are chasing, your career, or using your talents and skills to contribute to the greater good. Know that your purpose in life can change as you develop and age.
- **Fostering meaningful interpersonal connections** with others gives you a sense of belonging and helps you see that your existence brings positivity to the world. They tell

you, "You are here for a purpose." This message could be found in the positive impact on your family, friends, colleagues, romantic partners, and children.

- **Believing in a Higher Power** gives instant meaning to your life; knowing your faith is your significance. Your Creator made you for a reason, and you are put on this Earth to find your purpose. Your meaning in life is tied to your faith beliefs. Many people believe their purpose is to achieve a place in the afterlife.
- **Self-transcendence** allows you to experience life from a different perspective. Maslow's pyramid places self-actualization at the top. Experiences feel motivated by energies beyond the self. To experience self-transcendence, you need to reach self-actualization.

Therapists are specially trained to address and heal from trauma and manage shadow work. Life, wellness, and spiritual coaches typically do not work deeply with trauma healing but can be great resources for finding fulfillment and meaning in life.

WHY WE NEED HOPE AND HOW TO CREATE IT

Hope provides a reason to keep going, no matter the circumstances. Hope is defined as expecting something that will happen in your favor. Let's say you have set a goal. You put in effort to achieve it, which makes you wake up every day excited to get closer and closer to your goal because you are hopeful.

Hope is significant because it makes you braver, happier, and less stressed. We sometimes take the aspect of being optimistic for granted, but it can have a powerful impact on our quality of life. Being hopeful is believed to have a positive and healthy influence on your thoughts, behavior, and emotions. It can change your thought pattern from *I can't handle this,* to *I know I can get through it.* Your emotions can go from being worried and doubtful to being determined.

Being hopeful about the future has healing properties. Hope wins the battle against negative thoughts and demotivation, pulling you out of the darkness. Bring hope back into your life by creating it.

Here are some simple strategies to try:

- **Change your expectations** and set intentions for the day ahead for a brighter and happier mood.
- **Embrace a mindset** of hope and anticipation, allowing each day to unfold with delightful surprises. Remember, *"This too shall pass."* No life situation is permanent.
- **Find meaning** in the challenging seasons of life to teach you lessons and help you find the silver lining.
- **Be inspired and curious** by someone else's life story by asking a friend or family member about the most meaningful moment in their life.
- **Engage in activities** that help you feel centered and balanced. Usually, this means you've found balance in your body, mind, and spirit.
- **Add excitement** to your life by having a spontaneous day once a month.
- **Remember that the world** is a good place, and good humans still exist.
- **Live daily with the mindset** *"You only live once,"* and remove the spirit of stalling and postponing your dreams.

HOW TO ACHIEVE GOALS

Determine your values to successfully achieve your long-term goals related to your vision for healing from trauma. Values refer to the compass you use to navigate through life. Your values determine what you see as important. Your values are the rules and beliefs you strictly live by. Your values are always kept in the front row when making a decision. For example, if respect is crucial, you will consider ending a romantic connection once a man disrespects you.

Here is a list of some common values:

- Empathy
- Humility
- Kindness
- Altruism
- Loyalty
- Attentiveness
- Respect
- Integrity
- Honesty
- Generosity

Values help you set boundaries, reach your goals, and create the future you envision for yourself. Start aligning your life more closely with your values. Acknowledge that it's a continuous daily work in progress to ensure your life is congruent with your values. Practice introspection often, be present in the moment, and live committed to your values. By doing this, you will achieve life experiences that bring you inner peace, satisfaction, and success.

INTERACTIVE ELEMENT

The Free Interactive Elements Workbook for Chapter 9 provides instructions for Creating a Vision Board to represent your future healing goals. It also includes additional resources for gathering information for the vision board.

SEGUE

The final chapter will help you build a solid foundation for your future now that you can influence your vision of a better life.

10

BUILDING ON YOUR FOUNDATIONS

When we tackle obstacles, we find hidden reserves of
courage and resilience we did not know we had. And it
is only when we are faced with failure do we realize
that these resources were always there within us. We
only need to find them and move on with our lives.

— A. P. J. ABDUL KALAM

When you experience a traumatic event, you become aware of the skills and resources you already have within you. You might be surprised at how well you handled a situation or by certain traits you used to overcome a tough time. This awareness means that everything you need is already within you. All you have to do is increase your self-awareness, get to know yourself better, and hone your skills. You were born with the foundation to handle life and everything that will be thrown at you in the future. You can sharpen your skills and build on your foundation.

Let's review the story of Jo, a trauma survivor:

Jo had known George for approximately a year. They first crossed paths at a restaurant where he worked when he caught her attention during a lackluster date. Jo reminisced, "My date was too engrossed in a sports game, so George initiated a conversation and even offered me a free drink. Despite the bad date, the restaurant became my go-to place." Their interactions at the restaurant started friendly, with hugs, chats, and friendly kisses on the cheek.

As time passed, George's behavior took a turn for the worse. Jo noticed his frustration when she arrived on other dates, and he occasionally caused scenes when she conversed with the bartender. Jo recalled confronting him about his unwarranted reactions, firmly stating that he had no right to be upset. George later apologized and officially asked her out, coinciding with the end of another romantic disappointment in Jo's life.

Their dates were initially platonic, and Jo set clear boundaries as George expressed interest in a more intimate connection. "I wanted to take things very slow and didn't want to be physically intimate yet." George, expressing respect for her pace, assured her they would proceed at her comfort level. Jo found this sentiment sweet at the time.

Events took a chilling turn during a night out with a new friend. After consuming a few drinks at their usual spot, Jo experienced a blackout and woke up at home, unaware of what transpired. George claimed to have cared for her all night, and they exchanged seemingly ordinary texts the next day. But the truth unraveled when he sent a disturbing message expressing a desire for intimacy and revealing that they had sex.

Shocked and horrified, Jo confronted George, realizing that he had likely put something in her drink to cause the blackout and taken advantage of her intoxicated state. She recounted, "I told him on the phone, 'You knew I was drunk. I would have never been okay with that.'" The aftermath was emotionally devastating, with Jo seeking support from her advocate, best friend, and sister.

Not everyone in Jo's life responded with empathy. Two girlfriends blamed her and severed ties, while a close friend initially supported her but later turned accusatory. Jo embarked on a challenging journey of trauma therapy and support groups, facing obstacles in dealing with law enforcement.

The ultimate blow came when the state attorney declared, "We cannot press charges." Jo felt the justice system had failed her, leaving her story unvalidated, feeling like her empowerment and strength were snatched away. Jo found solace in her advocating sister's unwavering support despite these setbacks. "I wish the woman I first met in the hospital could see the strong woman you are now," her sister remarked, rekindling Jo's sense of empowerment.

George may have evaded legal consequences, but Jo remained resolute: "He cannot ever take away my power, my resilience, or my self-worth." To fellow survivors, Jo emphasized, "Even if the justice system fails us, or our friends don't believe us, it was NOT our fault, and we did NOT deserve it."

This chapter guides you into building a solid foundation for your future, including engaging in self-care and doing personal growth work.

THE SIGNIFICANCE OF BUILDING A SUPPORT NETWORK

To lean on your support network has been an overarching theme of the book. You have learned that having a support network helps you to be resilient and to support you through healing from trauma. Besides being wired for human connection, Maslow claims that after your physiological and safety needs are met, humans need to feel a sense of belonging. You crave to feel connected to others and be accepted. Lack of connection and choosing to isolate yourself may impede your healing. You need to satisfy those needs to develop self-esteem. Otherwise, you are blocking yourself from building confidence and reaching your potential.

Research has proven that having a support network of people with whom you share strong bonds is essential to balance your mental health. Although having at least one supportive person in your life can do wonders, the research indicates that having more than three people in your support network is ideal. Having only one person to support you during hard times may exhaust that person. They may not always have the emotional and mental capacity or time to listen to you. In addition, having more than three people in your support network gives you various perspectives on your problem.

Note that different people in your life bring out different sides of you. For example, you may be open, honest, and able to cry with your friend, while you cannot be completely vulnerable with your sister. One person may be the serious friend who gives you direct but great advice, while the other is funny and light-hearted, treats you with empathy, and comforts you. Varying perspectives offer multiple options.

Tips to Expand Your Support Network

A more extensive support network is a benefit to heal from trauma. Here are ways to expand your support network:

- Build positive and healthy family relationships with intentional effort and energy.
- Evaluate the quality of your relationships with friends and whether including them in your support system is healthy.
- Join a small group in your faith community to find like-minded people who support your spiritual life.
- Befriend your work colleagues, and find out how your employer can support your mental health needs.
- Meet new people by attending community events and social gatherings.
- Find online groups that align with your interests and the situation you are going through.
- Become involved in local events in your community.

Choose people with empathic, supportive, and trustworthy qualities to be part of your support network. Note that to build strong relationships with others, you must show the characteristics you want to see in others. Care about your family, friends, and mentors by asking about their challenges. Remember, to have a friend, you must be a friend. So, offer your support and love where you can.

THE RELATIONSHIP BETWEEN SELF-CARE AND HEALING

Self-care is often portrayed in the media as a luxurious and indulgent activity. However, in mental health, self-care refers to an individualized plan encompassing various domains of one's life, such as physical, emotional, social, professional, financial, and spiritual. Caring for yourself can solve many problems and identify neglected areas of life.

Self-care can even help individuals to understand why they are unable to move past trauma. It acts as a soothing balm that makes life easier and smoother, ultimately enhancing the quality of one's life. Let's delve deeper into each self-care domain.

Physical Self-Care

Taking care of your physical self is essential for improving your well-being. You start to feel energized and more productive. Physical self-care involves having a healthy diet, exercising regularly, looking after your sleep hygiene, and scheduling regular check-ups with your doctor. Some ideas for enhancing your physical health are to sleep within an appropriate time frame for your body and ensure you are adequately hydrated, plan your meals in advance, eat protein at every meal, choose natural carbohydrates over processed food, and move your body at least 30 minutes daily. Hey, take the stairs instead of the elevator!

Mental Health Self-Care

Ensuring excellent mental health by engaging in mentally stimulating activities that exercise the mind. These activities offer health benefits by keeping you mentally fit and reducing the chances of developing degenerative diseases. Ideas to help you feel mentally stimulated could be enrolling in a new course, listening to interesting podcasts, solving puzzles, playing games, or reading a book.

Emotional Self-Care

Emotional self-care refers to processing and managing emotions and energizing yourself when you feel emotionally drained. It's all about having the tools to regulate your emotions and making healthy decisions to cope with overwhelming and intense emotions in the moment and later. Refer to Chapter 6, which discusses emotional triggers and provides various strategies to manage your emotional well-being.

Social Self-Care

Taking care of the social domain in your life focuses on satisfying your social needs. Social self-care involves nurturing the relationships you currently have in your life by spending quality time with loved ones. Consider your emotional and mental capacity to spend time with others. Your social battery may run out after spending even a short time with particular family or friends. To take care of your social needs, go on lunch dates, accept invitations to social gatherings, or do video calls with friends and family. It's also good to reconnect with people you haven't seen recently.

Professional Self-Care

What does your professional life look like, and how does it make you feel? Pursuing a career or education can often be overwhelming and highly stressful. You may feel burned out trying to juggle and cope with everything simultaneously. Such stress can lead to unhealthy sleeping patterns, poor dietary habits, and difficulty regulating emotions. To alleviate stress, set achievable goals, practice good time management, delegate tasks if necessary, and set boundaries.

Financial Self-Care

As an adult, you might wish to return to being a child when finances were not a worry. Money is a common source of stress that creates a struggle for many of us. Life is getting more expensive as years go by. Sometimes, you may only have enough money to last from month to month. Other times, you have to cut down on specific areas of your life to have enough to cover bare necessities. Taking control of your finances can alleviate anxiety and make life less stressful. You can find enhanced control by creating a monthly budget, having financial goals, and living a lifestyle that matches your income.

Spiritual Self-Care

Many individuals turn to spiritual and religious avenues for solace, empowerment, and guidance. Spiritual self-care involves addressing your faith needs, participating in spiritual activities that bring you a sense of fulfillment, and seeking answers to life's profound questions that only your faith practice can provide. Some methods to attain spiritual fulfillment encompass prayer, meditation, immersing oneself in nature, and participating in sacred or spiritual gatherings or services.

How to Include Self-Care in Your Everyday Routine

Knowing each type of self-care domain is one thing, but implementing self-care practices in your life is another. Trauma survivors may find it uncomfortable to practice self-care at first, as they believe they don't need or deserve it. Start small and do what makes you feel comfortable as you start a self-care routine.

Use these five steps to help you begin your self-care routine:

1. Start by writing down everything that makes you happy, safe, and centered.
2. Consider including the things you wrote down in Step 1 into your daily routine.
3. Establish goals for the self-care practices you wish to incorporate into your daily routine.
4. Celebrate your progress and achievements.
5. Adjust and change your self-care plan as you move forward.

Self-care is a vital part of your daily life because it promotes physical health, prevents you from developing certain illnesses and diseases, and aids in managing stress. A self-care plan is an answer to address many problems.

HOW TO INCREASE PERSONAL GROWTH

When you stop learning, you stop growing.

— KENNETH H. BLANCHARD

A large part of healing is focused on self-improvement and personal growth. Achieving personal growth is changing bad habits, destructive behaviors, and reactions to life. Personal growth can occur naturally, especially after going through a dark time. Still, it can also be achieved by intentionally improving yourself.

Personal growth is unlearning everything that spirals your well-being and learning new skills and behaviors that enhance your chances of becoming a better version of yourself. To achieve personal development, you must feel motivated, desire to better yourself, and be open to change.

An honest and unbiased analysis during introspection is essential to improve yourself. This process is a way to find your weaknesses, toxic behaviors, and self-sabotaging habits. When you list them, you will know where to start and what to work on for self-improvement.

Here are some opportunities to achieve personal growth:

- Recognize your strengths.
- Set personal goals for yourself.
- Cultivate a positive mindset.
- Educate yourself on topics that offer new insight.
- Ask a trusted supporter to be your mentor.

Personal growth requires you to step out of your comfort zone and do things you may find uncomfortable. However, these will ultimately benefit you as growth happens in those gaps.

> *Courage is very important. Like a muscle, it is strengthened by use.*
>
> — RUTH GORDON

Let the quote inspire you to embrace unfamiliar experiences. The more you do, the less frightening they will be and the more you can grow.

INTERACTIVE ELEMENT

The Chapter 10 Interactive Element provides a Self-Assessment Tool to evaluate your current self-care practices and identify areas for improvement. If you haven't downloaded the Free Interactive Elements Workbook, scan the QR Code to access it.

SEGUE

You made it through the tough stuff! Now, with your solid foundation, let's pull it all together in the conclusion.

CONCLUSION

> *Then, one day, it clicks. The pain you had turns into peace as you accept that everything had to happen exactly as it did for you to be exactly who you are now. You hold no blame, bitterness, or resentment toward the experience, person, or yourself. Instead, you see it as the catalyst that led to your change and development. The very storm that shook so much in you also worked to clear your path.*

— MORGAN RICHARD OLIVIER

Nurture Emotional Well-Being for Women is about processing the past to move on and heal the emotional wounds you have been carrying. This book aims to lighten your load by teaching you emotional regulation skills and resilience so you can be an empowered individual. I encourage you to get up after being knocked down and learn ways to drag yourself out of the bottomless, dark pit of trauma symptoms and emotional triggers. I hope this book has prepared you to embark on your healing journey. You already have everything you need within you.

Success and healing can be found after surviving trauma. In the entourage of human experiences, stories of pain and resilience weave together, creating a complex narrative across diverse backgrounds. Becky's journey traces its roots to her tumultuous childhood, where navigating her mother's mental illness left her walking on fragile eggshells. Deprived of parental nurturing, Becky, the eldest among her siblings, found herself shouldering the responsibilities of caring for herself and household management.

Becky's life took an unexpected turn as an adult with the betrayal of her high school sweetheart, leading to the dissolution of their marriage. The aftermath of this heart-wrenching experience demanded strenuous efforts for emotional healing. Guided by her unwavering faith, Becky learned that humans are prone to falter. She realized that harboring resentment only obstructs the way to inner peace. She moves forward with the love and support of her current husband.

Becky now faces a new chapter of adversity with a breast cancer diagnosis. She is fortunate to have had a successful response to chemotherapy. Along with a double mastectomy and ongoing hormone suppressant medication, Becky is cancer-free. The experience was physically demanding, and now, two years later, she feels physically healed. So, why do upcoming scans bring her to the brink of a panic attack?

Recalling the memory of her scan, she recounts, "The date of my last scan was particularly challenging. However, the results provided relief—the scan was clear, and my blood work displayed positive indicators." Despite these moments of triumph, Becky remains acutely aware of the ongoing emotional hurdles accompanying her journey toward complete healing.

Breast cancer becomes a transformative journey, etching its mark on Becky's body, mind, and spirit. The journey toward emotional healing unfolds as a marathon, demanding resilience and introspection. Triggered by discussions of the cancer experiences of others, Becky grapples with her impending oncology visits and upcoming scans.

In this ongoing healing journey, Becky can discover the art of expecting positivity by relinquishing undue stress over uncertain futures. Embracing control over controllable aspects becomes her anchor, fostering equilibrium amid life's uncertainties.

Becky recognizes forgiveness as a powerful tool for healing emotional wounds. It doesn't mean condoning or excusing someone's actions but instead releasing the hold that anger and resentment have on her. Forgiving others can free her from carrying the weight of past grievances. Forgiveness is a choice.

Often overlooked but equally crucial is forgiving ourselves. Self-forgiveness is about letting go of self-blame and self-judgment. Forgiveness emerges as a profound choice and practice, a key to dismantling roadblocks and liberating oneself from the shackles of the past. Forgiveness intertwines with resilience, guiding Becky toward a brighter, self-affirming future. As we reach the end of this transformative journey through the pages of *Nurture Emotional Well-Being for Women*, I want to leave you with a powerful call to action—a roadmap to continue your path to healing and self-discovery.

- **Embrace your journey:** Recognize that healing from trauma is lifelong. Accept the ups and downs, knowing each step forward is a victory.
- **Seek support:** Healing is not a solitary endeavor. Contact therapists, coaches, support groups, and trusted friends or family members who can provide guidance, understanding, and a listening ear.
- **Practice self-compassion:** Be kind to yourself. Understand that healing is not a linear process, and setbacks are a natural part of growth. Treat yourself with the same compassion you would offer to a dear friend.
- **Set and pursue your goals:** Take the time to define your goals and intentions for the future. Set actionable steps to move closer to creating a better version of yourself.
- **Prioritize self-care:** Make self-care a non-negotiable part of your daily routine. Whether meditation, exercise, journaling, or spending time in nature, commit to nurturing your well-being.
- **Stay curious and educated:** Explore resources, books, and workshops that resonate with your healing journey. Knowledge is a powerful tool on the path to recovery.
- **Advocate for others:** If you feel comfortable, share your story and insights with others who may be struggling. Your experiences and resilience can inspire and support fellow survivors.
- **Celebrate your progress:** Your achievements, no matter how small, are a testament to your strength and determination.
- **Stay open to growth:** Be open to new experiences, relationships, and opportunities for personal growth. Healing allows you to live a life filled with purpose and fulfillment.

- **Remember your power:** Never forget the power within you—the strength that brought you this far. You can shape your destiny and create a future filled with joy and purpose.

This book can serve as a valuable guide, but remember, your journey is uniquely yours. You possess incredible resilience and power, capable of healing, growing, and thriving beyond your wildest dreams. Embrace your path and believe in your ability to create a fulfilling and prosperous future. It's time to step into your power and live a life reflecting your strength and potential.

I'm cheering you on!

Terri Sterk

tsterkemotionalhealing@gmail.com

LEAVE A REVIEW!

Now that you have everything you need to empower your recovery after trauma, build lasting resilience, and transform pain into strength, it's time to pass on your new knowledge and show other readers where they can find the same help.

Leaving your honest opinion of this book on Amazon and Audible will show other women where they can find the information they want and pass on your passion for emotional well-being.

Use this QR Code to access the review link and leave your review.

Note: Use your applicable country's Amazon site for those outside the USA.

Thank you for your help. Emotional well-being is kept alive when we pass on our knowledge – and you're helping to do just that.

Please leave an honest review on Amazon if this book helped you acquire the skills and tools to overcome your past trauma.

Your honest review will mean the world to me!

I'm cheering you on!

Terri Sterk

REFERENCES

Abdul Kalam, A. P. J. (n.d.). *A. P. J. Abdul Kalam quotes*. Brainy Quote. https://www.brainyquote.com/quotes/a_p_j_abdul_kalam_589755

Ackerman, C. E. (2017). *Cognitive distortions: 22 examples & worksheets (& PDF)*. PositivePsychology.com. https://positivepsychology.com/cognitive-distortions/

Ackerman, C. E. (2018). *What is self-worth & how do we build it? (incl. worksheets)*. PositivePsychology.com. https://positivepsychology.com/self-worth/

After Trauma (n.d.). *Grace's story*. https://www.aftertrauma.org/survivors-stories/graces-story#:~:text=I%20set%20myself%20a%20new,I%20couldn%27t%20use%20it.

American Psychological Association (n.d.). *What is posttraumatic stress disorder (PTSD)?* https://www.psychiatry.org/patients-families/ptsd/what-is-ptsd#

Angelou, M. (n.d.). *Maya Angelou quotes*. Brainy Quote. https://www.brainyquote.com/quotes/maya_angelou_634505

Bennett, T. (2019). *Memory distortion is real: Here's why your brain creates false or distorted memories*. Thrive Works. https://thriveworks.com/blog/memory-distortion/

Better Health Channel (n.d.). *Trauma and families*. https://www.betterhealth.vic.gov.au/health/healthyliving/trauma-and-families

Black, E. (2020). *Emotions are messengers*. https://townsvillepsychologist.com.au/emotions-are-messengers/#:~

Bradshaw, F. (2018). *7 ways to keep going when you want to give up*. Mind Tools. https://www.mindtools.com/blog/7-ways-keep-going/

Braich, A. S. (2023). *The connection between trauma and dysregulation*. Camino Recovery. https://www.caminorecovery.com/blog/the-connection-between-trauma-and-dysregulation/

Burton, M. S., Cooper, A. A., Feeny, N. C. and Zoellner, L. A. (2015). The enhancement of natural resilience in trauma interventions. *Journal of Contemporary Psychotherapy*. *45*(4), 193–204. https://www.linkedin.com/pulse/resilient-entrepreneur-inspiring-stories-overcoming-success-de-knoop/

Cafasso, J. (2023). *Traumatic Events*. Healthline. https://www.healthline.com/health/traumatic-events

Caramela, S. (2023). *How to tell your loved ones about your trauma*. Healthy Place. https://www.healthyplace.com/blogs/traumaptsdblog/2023/7/how-to-tell-your-loved-ones-about-your-trauma

Casabianca, S. S. (2022). *15 cognitive distortions to blame for negative thinking.* PsychCentral. https://psychcentral.com/lib/cognitive-distortions-negative-thinking

Cherry, K. (2023). *Toxic positivity—why it's harmful and what to say instead.* verywellmind. https://www.verywellmind.com/what-is-toxic-positivity-5093958

Chowdhury, M. R. (2019). *What is emotional resilience? (+six proven ways to build It).* PositivePsychology.com. https://positivepsychology.com/emotional-resilience/

Coller, N. (2013). *Why your thoughts are not real.* Psychology Today. https://www.psychologytoday.com/intl/blog/inviting-monkey-tea/201308/why-your-thoughts-are-not-real

Collier, L. (2016). Growth after trauma: Why are some people more resilient than others—and can it be taught? *American Psychological Association, 47*(10), 48. https://www.apa.org/monitor/2016/11/growth-trauma

Cooks-Campbell, A. (2023). *How inner child work enables healing and playful discovery.* Better Up. https://www.betterup.com/blog/inner-child-work

Cooks-Campbell, A. (2023). *Triggered? Learn what emotional triggers are and how to deal with them.* Better Up. https://www.betterup.com/blog/triggers

Cutruzulla, K. (2018). *How to be more hopeful.* Ideas.ted.com. https://ideas.ted.com/how-to-be-more-hopeful/

Dhrymes, J. (n.d.). *Trauma self-assessment quiz.* Dr. Jim Dhrymes. https://drdhrymes.com/trauma-self-assessment-quiz/

Dr. Whitney (n.d.). *Visualization for greater clarity: Aligning with your true desires.* Dr. Whitney. https://whitneygordon-mead.com/2021/07/20/visualization-for-greater-clarity-aligning-with-your-true-desires/

Earnshaw, E. (2019). *The power of your personal narrative.* A Better Life Therapy. https://abetterlifetherapy.com/blog/the-power-of-your-personal-narrative

Emory University (n.d.). *Self-advocacy and resiliency: Essential traits for women in leadership roles.* https://ece.emory.edu/articles-news/self-advocacy-and-resiliency.php

Emotional Resolution With Cedric Bertelli (n.d.). *Success stories…many more stories HERE.* https://www.cedricbertelli.com/success-stories

Equipping Godly Women. (n.d.). Christian Self-Care: What the Bible Says About Self-Care. Retrieved March 19, 2024, from https://equippinggodlywomen.com/faith/christian-self-care/

Expressions Counselling (n.d.). *Our narrative therapy case studies and success stories.* https://expressionscounselling.com/narrative-therapy-case-study/

Finch, J. (2019). *How do I know if I've been affected by trauma?* Centre for Clinical Psychology. https://ccp.net.au/how-do-i-know-if-ive-been-affected-by-trauma/

Forbes (2020). *Five steps women can take to self-advocate.* https://www.forbes.com/sites/ellevate/2020/08/25/five-steps-women-can-take-to-self-advocate/?sh=bb6776d7d56f

Gilette, H. (2021). *Main signs of childhood trauma in children and adults.* PsychCentral. https://psychcentral.com/ptsd/effects-and-signs-of-childhood-trauma#whats-trauma

Gillette, H. (2022). *7 evidence-based strategies to manage emotional pain.* PsychCentral. https://psychcentral.com/blog/how-to-deal-with-emotional-pain

Gillihan, S.J. (2019). *The healing power of telling your trauma story.* Psychology Today. https://www.psychologytoday.com/za/blog/think-act-be/201903/the-healing-power-telling-your-trauma-story

Gillis, K. (2019). *5 mental health goals for trauma survivors in the new year.* Psychology Today. https://www.psychologytoday.com/za/blog/invisible-bruises/202112/5-mental-health-goals-trauma-survivors-in-the-new-year

Goldsmith, O. (n.d.). *Oliver Goldsmith quotes.* https://www.brainyquote.com/quotes/oliver_goldsmith_383305

Grinspoon, P. (2022). *How to recognize and tame your cognitive distortions.* Harvard Health Publishing. https://www.health.harvard.edu/blog/how-to-recognize-and-tame-your-cognitive-distortions-202205042738

Gupta, S. (2023). *How to improve your self-worth and why it's important.* verywellmind. https://www.verywellmind.com/what-is-self-worth-6543764

Gupta, S. (2023). *What is unresolved trauma?* verywellmind. https://www.verywellmind.com/unresolved-trauma-symptoms-causes-diagnosis-and-treatment-6753365

Hailey, L. (n.d.). *How to set boundaries: 5 ways to draw the line politely.* Science of People. https://www.scienceofpeople.com/how-to-set-boundaries/

Handson, H. (2016). *10 resiliency building skills to practice to make progress in trauma recovery.* New Synapse. https://www.new-synapse.com/aps/wordpress/?p=1825

Health Match (2022). *A guide to the five stages of trauma.* https://healthmatch.io/ptsd/5-stages-of-trauma

Holt, T. (2020). *A story of trauma and resilience.* Paces Connection. https://www.pacesconnection.com/blog/a-story-of-trauma-and-resilience

Indeed (2023). *5 areas of personal growth (plus tips for development).* https://www.indeed.com/career-advice/career-development/areas-of-personal-growth

Jo (2023). *Jo's story.* The Survivors Trust. https://www.thesurvivorstrust.org/blog/jos-story

Johnson, K. (n.d.). *Breaking like glass: A story of complex trauma and healing.* OC87 Recovery Diaries. https://oc87recoverydiaries.org/complex-trauma-and-healing/

Josefowitz, N. (2021). *3 steps to identify what triggers you.* Psychology Today. https://www.psychologytoday.com/za/blog/cbt-made-simple/202103/3-steps-identify-what-triggers-you

Klynn, B. (2021). *Emotional regulation: Skills, exercises, and strategies.* Better Up. https://www.betterup.com/blog/emotional-regulation-skills

Lawler, M. (2022). *How to start a self-care routine you'll follow.* Everyday Health. https://www.everydayhealth.com/self-care/start-a-self-care-routine/

Lebow, H. l. (2021). *Trauma denial: How to recognize it and why it matters.* Psych-Central. https://psychcentral.com/blog/denial-of-trauma-signs

Lennon, A. (2022). *How and why finding meaning in life can improve well-being.* Medical News Times. https://www.medicalnewstoday.com/articles/how-and-why-finding-meaning-in-life-can-improve-well-being

Leonard, J. (2020). *What is trauma.uma? What to know.* Medical News Today. https://www.medicalnewstoday.com/articles/trauma#definition

Levine, P. A. (n.d.). *Trauma quotes.* Brainy Quote. https://www.brainyquote.com/quotes/peter_a_levine_864302?src=t_trauma

Levine, P. A. (n.d.). *Trauma quotes.* Brainy Quote. https://www.brainyquote.com/quotes/peter_a_levine_864300?src=t_trauma

Lindberg, S. (2023). *How to let go of things from the past.* Healthline. https://www.healthline.com/health/how-to-let-go

Madly Calm (n.d.). *Success stories.* https://www.madlycalm.com/testimonials

Manitoba Trauma Information and Education Centre (n.d.). *Phases of trauma.* https://trauma-informed.ca/recovery/phases-of-trauma-recovery/#:~:

Marie, S. (2021). *How to reduce anxiety right here, right now.* PsychCentral. https://psychcentral.com/anxiety/how-to-reduce-anxiety-quickly#long-term-changes

MHA (n.d.). *Helpful vs harmful: Ways to manage emotions.* https://www.mhanational.org/helpful-vs-harmful-ways-manage-emotions

Mind (2023). *Trauma.* https://www.mind.org.uk/information-support/types-of-mental-health-problems/trauma/about-trauma/

Mitts, C. (n.d.). *12 very common examples of trauma.* Ipseity Counselling. https://ipseitycounselingclinic.com/2019/09/03/examples-of-trauma/

Nesenoff, A. (2020). *Five Ways to tell if you are suffering from underlying trauma.* Tikvah Lake. https://www.tikvahlake.com/blog/five-ways-to-tell-if-you-are-suffering-from-underlying-trauma/

NHS (n.d.). *Complex PTSD - Post-traumatic stress disorder.* https://www.nhs.uk/mental-health/conditions/post-traumatic-stress-disorder-ptsd/complex/

Nightingale, E. (n.d.). *Earl Nightingale quotes.* Brainy Quote. https://www.brainyquote.com/quotes/earl_nightingale_390812

Nir and Far (n.d.). *A list of 20 values [and why people can't agree on more].* https://www.nirandfar.com/common-values/

Not Salmon (n.d.). *15 quotes about emotionally healing from trauma and challenges.* https://www.notsalmon.com/2016/04/11/quotes-emotionally-heal/

Parker, S. (2023). *Four ways we avoid our feelings—and what to do instead.* Greater Good Magazine. https://greatergood.berkeley.edu/article/item/four_ways_we_avoid_our_feelings_and_what_to_do_instead

Perry, E. (2022). *The benefits of shadow work and how to use it in your journey.* Better Up. https://www.betterup.com/blog/shadow-work

Psychology Today (n.d.). *Post-traumatic growth.* https://www.psychologytoday.com/za/basics/post-traumatic-growth

Rainn (n.d.). *Courageous's story.* https://www.rainn.org/survivor-stories/courageous%E2%80%99s-story

Rainn (n.d.). Kim's story. https://www.rainn.org/survivor-stories/kim%E2%80%99s-story

Ramirez-Duran, D. (2020). *Somatic experiencing therapy: 10 best exercises & examples.* PositivePsychology.com. https://positivepsychology.com/somatic-experiencing/

Raypole, C. (2020). *How to identify and manage your emotional triggers.* Healthline. https://www.healthline.com/health/mental-health/emotional-triggers

Regan, S. (2023). *The value of shadow work + 3 exercises to get started, from mental health professionals.* mbgmindfulness. https://www.mindbodygreen.com/articles/what-is-shadow-work

SAMHSA (2023). *Recognizing and treating child traumatic stress.* https://www.samhsa.gov/child-trauma/recognizing-and-treating-child-traumatic-stress#:~:text=Traumatic%20events%20may%20include%3A,or%20experiencing%20intimate%20partner%20violence

Saxena, S. (2023). *Narrative therapy: How it works & what to expect.* Choosing Therapy. https://www.choosingtherapy.com/narrative-therapy/

Shamanic Healing of Ames (n.d.). *What are your intentions for healing?* https://shamanichealingofames.com/2018/12/15/what-are-your-intentions-for-healing/

Suicide Call Back Service (n.d.). *How to build a strong support network.* https://www.suicidecallbackservice.org.au/mental-health/how-to-build-a-strong-support-network/

Survivor's Guilt: Definition, Symptoms, Traits, Causes, Treatment. (n.d.) Verywell Mind. https://www.verywellmind.com/survivors-guilt-4688743

Swain, K. D., Pillay, B. J. & Kliewer, W. (2017). Traumatic stress and psychological functioning in a South African adolescent community sample. *South African Journal of Psychiatry,* pp. 23, 1008. https://www.ncbi.nlm.nih.gov/pmc/articles/PMC6138196/

The Guest House (2022). *The benefits of processing your trauma.* https://www.theguesthouseocala.com/the-benefits-of-processing-your-trauma/#:~

Trauma Survivor's Network (n.d.). *Dawne's story.* https://www.traumasurvivorsnetwork.org/pages/1174

Turkel, L. (2023). *37 calm quotes that will bring you inner peace.* Reader's Digest. https://www.rd.com/list/quotes-calm/

Tzu, L. (n.d.). *Lao Tzu quotes.* Brainy Quote. https://www.brainyquote.com/quotes/

lao_tzu_130742

US. Department of Veterans Affairs (n.d.). *PTSD: National Center for PTSD.* https://www.ptsd.va.gov/professional/treat/specific/ptsd_research_women.asp

Van Edwards, V. (n.d.). *6 effective tips to politely say no (that actually work!).* Science of People. https://www.scienceofpeople.com/how-to-say-no/

Virginia Commonwealth University (2023). *7 types of self-care and why you should practice them.* https://onlinesocialwork.vcu.edu/blog/types-of-self-care/

VitalWorkLife. (2020.). Engage in the 5 pillars of resilience during tough times. https://insights.vitalworklife.com/engage-in-the-5-pillars-of-resilience-during-tough-times

Webb, J. (2023). *A closer look at the 35 most commonly felt emotions... and the emotional confusion of the neglected.* Psychology Today. https://www.psychology today.com/us/blog/childhood-emotional-neglect/202303/35-commonly-felt-emotions-and-what-they-mean#:~:Well+Good. (2023). How to Live Longer, According to a Holistic Medicine Specialist. Retrieved March 19, 2024, from https://www.wellandgood.com/holistic-medicine-specialist-longevity/

Wilder Research (2014). *Trauma and resilience.* https://www.wilder.org/sites/default/files/imports/AnokaCountyMWCtrauma%20Snapshot_10-14.pdf

Women Against Abuse (n.d.). *Jamie's Story: Jamie shared her story at the 2019 iPledge Campaign press conference.* https://www.womenagainstabuse.org/stories/jamies-story

.

Milton Keynes UK
Ingram Content Group UK Ltd.
UKHW022332041224
452010UK00019B/1125